Yoga and Nature, My Life 1

Seungyong Lee's Essays on Yoga and Meditation

Seungyong Lee's Essays on Yoga and Meditation
Yoga and Nature, My Life I

Published in the Republic of Korea by Hongik Yoga Institute
Nae-aneui Ddeul, 19 Jodonhandaengi-gil, Chungju-si,
Dongryang-myeon, Chungcheongbuk-do
Telephone: Seoul office 82-2-333-2350
Fax: Seoul office 82-2-333-2351
Homepage: http://www.yogahi.com

Copyright © 2014, Seungyong Lee
All rights reserved under International Copyright Conventions. No part of this book may be reproduced in any form, or by anymeans, electronic or mechanical, including photocopying, unless specifically permitted in the text or by written permission from the copyright owner.

ISBN 978-89-86748-22-2 04690
ISBN 978-89-86748-21-5 (SET)

Yoga and Nature, My Life 1

Hongik Yoga Institute

Recommendation

It seems people's lives that only headed outward are now coming inward. Though it is a small sign, it means a lot. Through this, we will rediscover a new way of life, which may be, at the same time, not new at all actually.

Sensual and materialistic lives didn't provide us with peace. It brought deficiency inside and expanded desires outside. In an infinitely busy life, we are losing ourselves and we are in conflict with others.

Like light coming through a narrow crack in a window, some teachers are guiding us to the inner world. They say that we should devote ourselves to practice and, only through practice, we can obtain peace. The practice they're saying is gradually coming as a topic of our time.

Now, many people are giving themselves up to work to find true self and spiritual enlightenment. This not only is in Korea but also spreads to the entire world. We can clearly see that westerners are heading to countries like Nepal and Bhutan where there is rich spiritual and religious heritage and flourishing culture historically with well-preserved natural and living environment on a relatively pure civilization even though people there are not enjoying material affluence. Heading inward is like going back home as it is getting dark. As we can take a rest only back home, practice is also a place to offer us true rest and peace.

This book presents a model for everyone who is willing to practice within their lives regardless of their gender, age or even religion. Not only does it show the author's life and process of practice over the past 20 years, but it also contains appearances of true practice from his young disciples. Advice for lives that the teacher gives to disciples and readers feels valuable as it inspires hope and confidence so that they think they also can do it.

Volume 1 introduces topics in life and his life story on how the author went into the path of practice and then shows contents of his lectures to change the concept of health and messages to disciples. In reading this book, a part for elucidating a true figure as a yoga teacher is not only applicable for yoga but for true leader figure in all areas of our society. Volume 2 conveys philosophical and ideological lessons easily which are related to yoga and our spirit in a form of letters and practice essays as if they were supposed to be sent to the general public. It is more interesting that pilgrimage essays are also included, which is rare for yoga books.

    The author has clarified that he would fulfill Hongik-Ingan and he is actually putting it into action. In addition, he well explains theoretically that yogic philosophy and indigenous Korean spirits are originally connected. His theories are unique but not excessive so it is possible to deeply and widely understand yoga through them. He also explains theories on natural health by using numerous examples in an interesting way, which makes people to easily apply them in their daily lives. I recommend anyone who has interest in health to read this.

    The author expresses equanimity as 'equability' and he always emphasizes it to disciples and people who learn yoga. Without the equability beyond any segregation, how else can we take the true path of life? Bodily health cannot be without mental fitness. When our mind is peaceful far from any segregation, we can naturally be healthy. He says "Yoga is consciousness-related exercise" as in Tao. Since yoga is not only bodily exercise but mental one, yoga cannot be anything but practice.

The teacher is a disciplinant so the path he walks on is peaceful and still. Those who are looking for the path can just walk with him. This book is the guide book for the path we take beside him. He courteously awakens us to how to treat our body and mind.

It is hard to meet a great teacher in life. You can find one with luck. This book is a gold mine in that sense. Practice hard with this book as if you dug gold out of the mine. Then you will get the gold of meeting up a great teacher.

November, 2551 as Buddha year (A.D. 2007)
Seong Jeon

*Seong Jeon: Abbot of Youngmunsa Temple, The Jogye Order of Korean Buddhism

Preface

Many people are traveling these days. In addition to famous sights and tourist attractions in Korea, they go literally everywhere like nearby Japan, China and Southeast Asia and even to Americas, Europe and Africa.

What we have to prepare for the trips is detailed information on the destination of the journey. In some cases, we sometimes need to ask directions to natives and receive help from them. Thanks to living in this information and internet era, we can explore paths and routes in the destination while sitting on a desk with books and searching information via internet.

No matter how convenient and quick the world is where we are living, however, it doesn't matter how many things we see in a short time to make it a good trip. I don't think that traveling seven European countries or America in a week or seeing Japan for three days is a true journey. It seems to be only for flying, taking some pictures and eating some foods several times that they've never tried before.

When we go on a trip, therefore, we need information and

guide for the destination and, depending on which path to take, what we see, hear and feel enormously varies. So do our lives.

There are so many different paths that we can take even in a single area. No matter which we choose, the choice is entirely ours. What matters is that, regardless of our choice, it does not end up as a personal issue but we are inevitably and closely connected with others, willingly or not. That is the fate of us living in this same period.

No matter which path we take, we should keep in mind that someone who is suggestible by others without a sense of purpose and sets off their way with subjective illusion or excessive bravado cannot finish their journey. To make something an end, there should have been start and process for the end. We human beings are also subject to the process of birth, life and death.

With people's increased interests in health, well-being and LOHAS since 2000s, yoga and meditation have become a big social issue. It is encouraging but it is worried to me who seek a natural life through yoga and meditation if haste would make waste. However good a thing is, a rapid boom cannot avoid side effects and it eventually has become a reality as the bubble in yoga burst since a few years ago. When it comes to yoga and meditation in a perspective of natural principles, it is somewhat weird to talk about so-called license. In some sense, the license can be necessary to give a minimum social guideline. As so many people thoughtlessly rush into yoga only after economical benefits, they hurt and get hurt one another.

There are many teachers educating yoga and meditation and students have various purposes in their learning as well. It doesn't matter you do yoga for a dietary purpose or good shape under any name like ○○ yoga or ○○ meditation. If any type of yoga cannot reach the essentials of yoga, however, it cannot be called true yoga but it is just an empty shell of the word yoga.

There are many paths to yoga based on thousands of years of its history. The paths, however, lead to one; Yoga is consciousness-related exercise. The core of yoga, as Yoga Sutra defines, is to remove restlessness of mind. Yoga is not just a physical exercise with bodily movements but is a question of how to keep and maximize purity and brightness of our consciousness through meditation. Therefore, philosophy of yoga asks how Atman, the personal consciousness, is combined with Brahman, the macrocosm.

Today, yoga has been rapidly expanded quantitatively and corresponding qualitative growth is also required. To those who truly love yoga with such a thirst, I sincerely hope this book would be a guide for a right path toward true yoga.

I want to express my gratitude to the director Heeju Lee and all teachers of Hongik Yoga Institute who have worked with me for manuscript proofreading through all summer and fall. I also give my thanks to Jihyun Choi for editorial design and staffs at Plan Field.

November, 2007
Seungyong Lee from Gab-bongjae

Preface for English Version

This book was published in 2007 November in Korea, which was for an affectionate suggestion from a Buddhist priest. The priest had already published several books then on his practice in Korea and made substantial contributions for popularization of Buddhism, hosting a radio broadcast.

One day, he and I talked about this and that and I came to tell him why I started yoga practice with interests in issues of life and death and what I had experienced while visiting many countries around the world and practicing yoga. After listening to my stories, he asked back.

"Why did you not write those good stories in a book? If I were you, I would have made several of them already. Moreover, Mr. Lee has such abundant and various spiritual experiences in practice beyond a religion with humane experience overcoming challenging health problems not as a monk but an ordinary person. It would be a good stimulus and precedent to many people who find 'practice in everyday life' only difficult if you let them know those experiences. Why don't you write them down in a book?"

Until then, I had never thought of writing a book with my very personal things but I started to think differently after that. If my experiences would be of a little help to those who are with difficult health problems, find yoga difficult and feel a thirst for spiritual issues, it would be to perform my mission just a bit in this world. Thus, this book came out to the world 7 years ago.

Couple of years ago, however, one of my foreign students who could speak and read Korean suggested translation for this book into English, saying that it would be very fresh to Westerners among other lots of books on yoga around the world and it would also be a good source to introduce and make them understand the diversity of yoga in Korea. Upon hearing that suggestion, I came to have hopes and expectations that what had been missed due to lack of smooth communication with foreign students could be made up for.

After all these stories, the book is published in English and ready to meet English-speaking readers. I hope this book would be helpful for readers around the world who are interested in yoga and meditation, natural health and life with practice. Lastly, I appreciate everyone sparing no efforts for publishing the book.

March 17th, 2014
Seungyong Lee

Seungyong Lee's Essays on Yoga and Meditation 1

Contents

Recommendation 5

Preface 9

Preface for English Version 13

Mother, My Lifelong Topic

· Hidden Virtue of Parents	22
· Babe in the Woods	27
· The Biggest Task in My Life	31
· Priest, Buddhism and Connection	37
· Four Pillars, Eight Characters and Schopenhauer	41
· Power of a Baked Sweet Potato	48
· Mother and Udambara	54
· Bongsun Sitting with Vajrasana	57

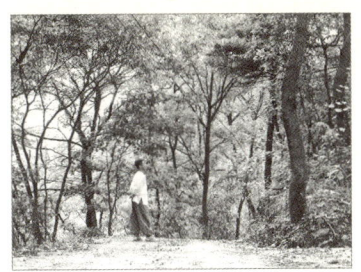

New Concept on Health

· Reinterpretation on Health	70
· Sources for Human Food are on Heaven and Earth	75
· When Stomach Meets Meat	89
· Mechanism of Cold and Cough	97
· Brilliantly	103
· Life Being Also of Principles of Screw	107
· Contemplation on Vitality	114
· Practice to be Exact and Practical	120
· Yoga, Trapped in Alternative Medicine	128

One Big Desire

· Let's Have One Big Desire　　　　　　　　　　　136
· Study to be Done in One's Youth　　　　　　　　141
· Where to Go After Using Up This Body　　　　　144
· Change Yourself　　　　　　　　　　　　　　　148
· Good Cause and Positive Mind　　　　　　　　　152
· Ought to Have Spiritual Pride　　　　　　　　　154
· Devotion only to Shine in Teaching Practice　　157
· Are You Guys Happy Now?　　　　　　　　　　160
· Katya's Visit to Korea
　 – Her Spiritual Hometown – after 10 Years　　165

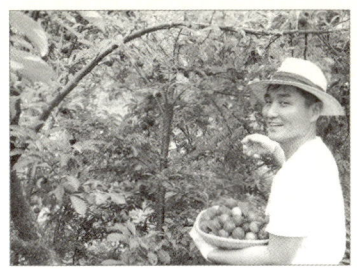

- The Rain of Your Teachings Still Wet in My Mind   170
- Letter from Poland   173
- An American potter came to Korea to learn Korean Onggi   176
- Nice and Calm Oasis of Mine   182
- The Spirit of my Yoga Master   185
- After the Hawaii Yoga Training   189
- After the Pilgrimage to Himalayas   192

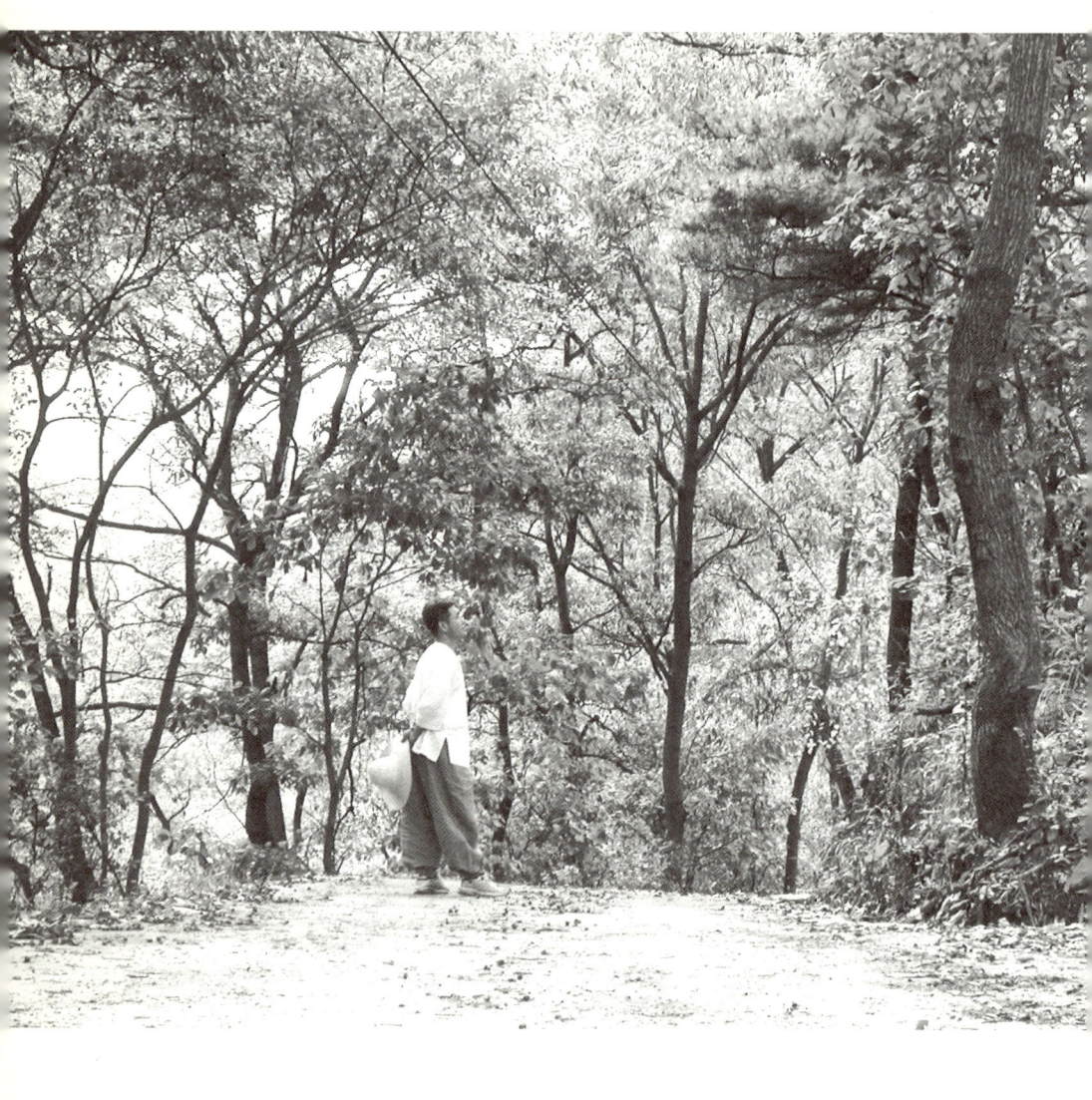

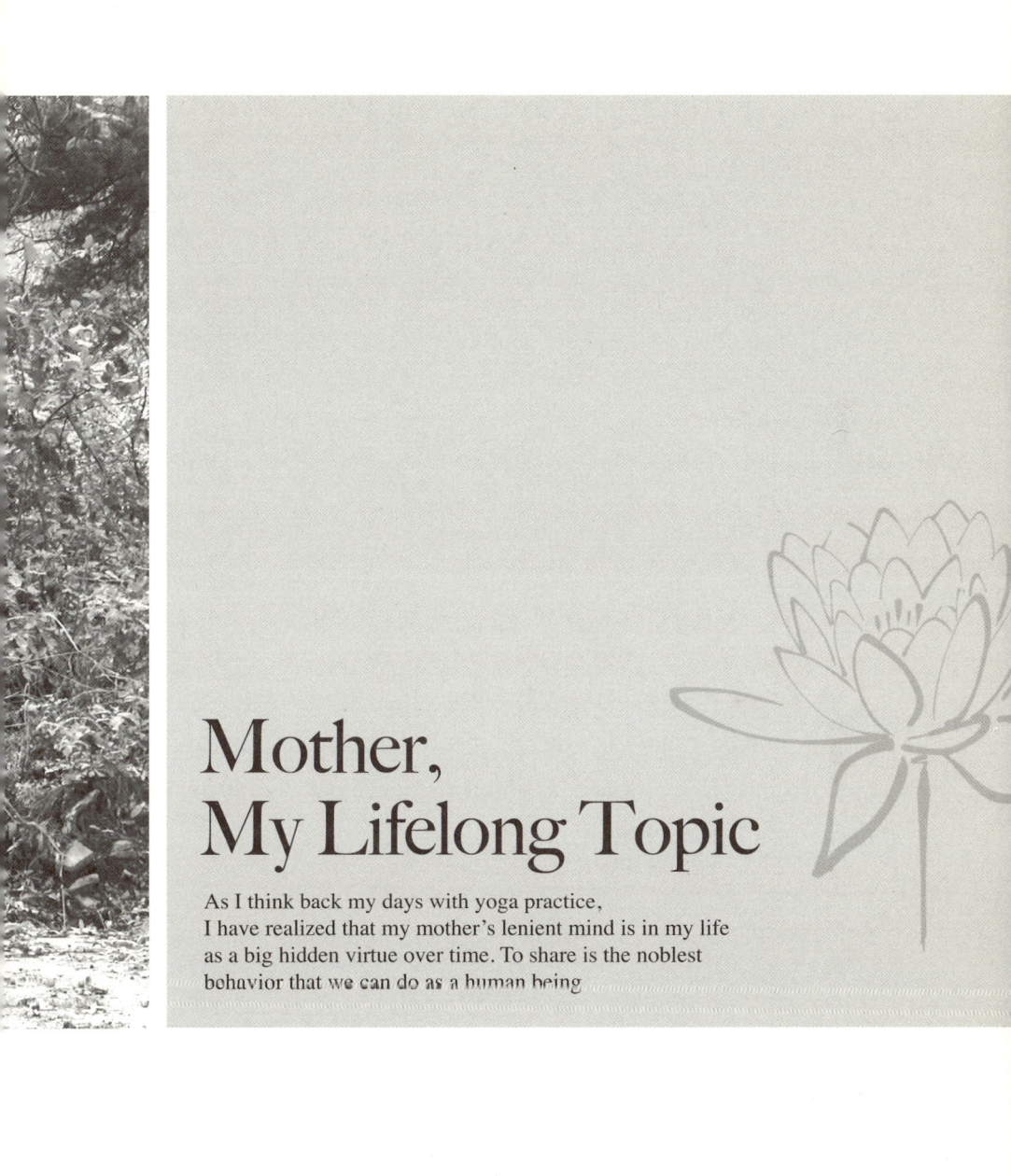

Mother, My Lifelong Topic

As I think back my days with yoga practice,
I have realized that my mother's lenient mind is in my life
as a big hidden virtue over time. To share is the noblest
behavior that we can do as a human being.

Hidden Virtue of Parents

That I have put emphasize on Hongik-Ingan[1] and my practice has been greatly inspired from our Korean national spirit is perhaps because my mother's life of sharing and mercy since my childhood has been deeply imprinted inside me.

When we made a digression after my lecture, someone asked me which days I would have picked if I had went back to past. I answered, without delay, that it would be childhood days I was with my mother.

As my parents said, I was an early riser when I was little. My

---

1) 'Hongik-Ingan' means extensively benefit all people

mother used to pray with scooping some water on the crocks every day while all my brothers and sisters were on their beds and only I was around her at such early dawn. They also said I was squatting down and scribbling on the ground throughout mother's prayer, I still have a faint memory of mother's back in prayer.

When mother said she would go to market early in the morning, I was milling around and rushing her as if I were waiting for it. It is still a fresh memory when I went to market with her. My mother used to get prepared by calling in a worker before going to market and the worker always showed up with a big handcart. It was common to calling in a worker and a handcart because transportation was not that varied back then. When the handcart arrived, I enjoyed traveling on it for market while humming a tune as if I were a triumphant general. The handcart was my own car on the way to market.

When coming back to home, the handcart was full of plump fruits and fresh vegetables like that of a fruit dealer. My mother never underbought fruits, like three or more watermelons and literally hundred oriental melons. Because there wasn't the refrigerator yet in 1960s, my mother washed the fruits and ran water into small and big buckets in a backyard to put them in. There was a low wooden bench at a corner of the yard and villagers and village elders used to sit round and stay on the bench at dusk talking about their daily lives. Whenever people were gathered, mother served them the fruits cut into big pieces from the early morning market. Then, my house was filled with laughter as if we had a big village feast. Even though I was just a child, I felt proud and happy that we had something to share with many others. It was especially enjoyable for me, such a slyboots, to go around with demilunar watermelon skin on my head like a helmet. During my childhood, I was in clover both materially and mentally with my mom.

Mother always loved to share things with neighbors and she was compassionate to anyone including lepers ^{they are now called patients with Hansen's disease} or beggars. In case of lepers, they were misunderstood that the disease was catching within the touch at that time so people would kick them out without even looking at them or drive them away soon with some food. Strangely, however, my mother never threw them out but set the table for them to sit down and take a rest for a while on a wooden bench under a grapevine beside the back door where people seldom used. I think she did that way every time out of her sympathy that they ate in hiding so that nobody would see them.

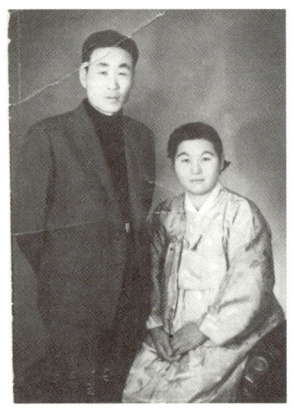

1963, My parent

I didn't know what that meant at that

time but as I think back my days with yoga practice, I have realized that my mother's lenient mind is in my life as a big hidden virtue over time. To share is the noblest behavior that we can do as a human being. The great inspiration on my practice is perhaps my mother's life of sharing and mercy since my childhood which has been deeply imprinted inside me.

My big sister who went to a university in Seoul[2] once bought me a pair of skates as a present. Thanks to the gift and mother's help, I could always win a game. Mother came to a rink and supported me whenever I had games. Unlike other mothers just watching from a distance, she cheered for me by coming into and going across the rink whenever I made a rotation and calling my name aloud. It would be the same for all mothers in the world but my mother totally devoted herself to her children. Wouldn't it be strange that I couldn't win the game with such support from mother?

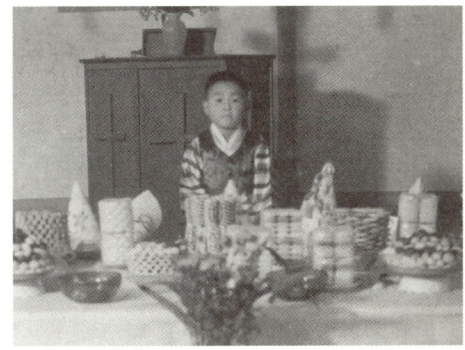
Birthday party in kindergarten

---

2) Capital city of South Korea

Mother, My Lifelong Topic

The system of one's consciousness is surely affected heavily from childhood experiences. Parental affection in one's childhood can be considered absolute in their life. People's personality is usually formed that time so it is unfortunate for a child to grow up without love from parents, not to grow up in poverty. There are people who went through underprivileged childhood and have a great personality sometimes but, in most cases, they cannot escape from complex on money even when they come to make huge money. So they don't know how to spend their money or they do spend only for showing it off. Even after those people make money, they don't have a broad mind or a concept of helping or being kind to others. Wouldn't it be that way and they feel anxious because they don't have experiences of hidden virtue in their lives?

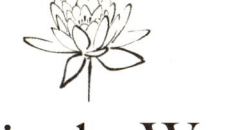

Babe in the Woods

I didn't know I had been a babe in the woods until then.

When I was a kid, it was even before Samsung[3] became such a conglomerate of today so Korea Electric Power Corporation was one of the largest scale enterprises that time. Considering the barley hump, I and my friends whose fathers were working in the power plant were relatively well-off. It was

---

3) Samsung(Group) is the largest South Korean multinational business conglomerate of South Korea.

natural for families that could afford their children's education to send them to study in Seoul during their junior high years or after graduating from junior high.

My family also moved to Seoul where my brothers and sisters were as soon as I finished junior high. My father bought a house with three bedrooms and a tiled kitchen floor in Ahyeon-dong, Seoul. The 'tiled kitchen' meant something in those days. Kitchen in Korean-style house in 1960s Seoul was almost on an earthen floor or a cement floor for richer families and then came the tiled kitchen.

My Seoul life, however, didn't go that much smoothly. Although it was the countryside, I was a boss of kids in the neighborhood and I was never behind in study or exercise compared to my friends. On the first exam after moving to Seoul, however, I placed 24th out of 72 students, which was way off an expectation that I would be, at least, in top five of the class. The number 24 was so strange and unfamiliar to me. New friends in Seoul said it was amazing for a bumpkin like me but

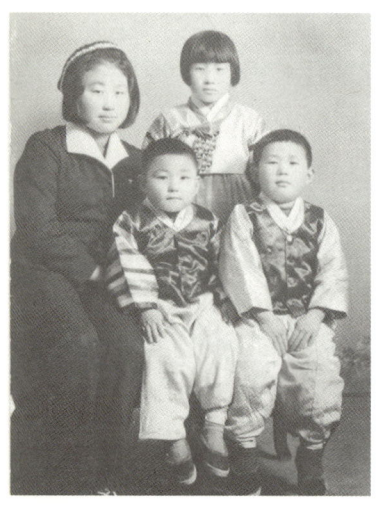

My oldest and second older sisters, I and second oldest brother (in the early 1960s)

it was shocking to me. One of my old friends moving to Seoul around the same time with me told me that he was just in the lower ranks on the first exam who now is a professor at Seoul National University after all the hard work.

 I didn't know I had been a babe in the woods until then. Seoul was the city where people from all over the country with various backgrounds came over and where those people competed with each other. Everything that was special back in my hometown became usual things for people including me after moving to Seoul.

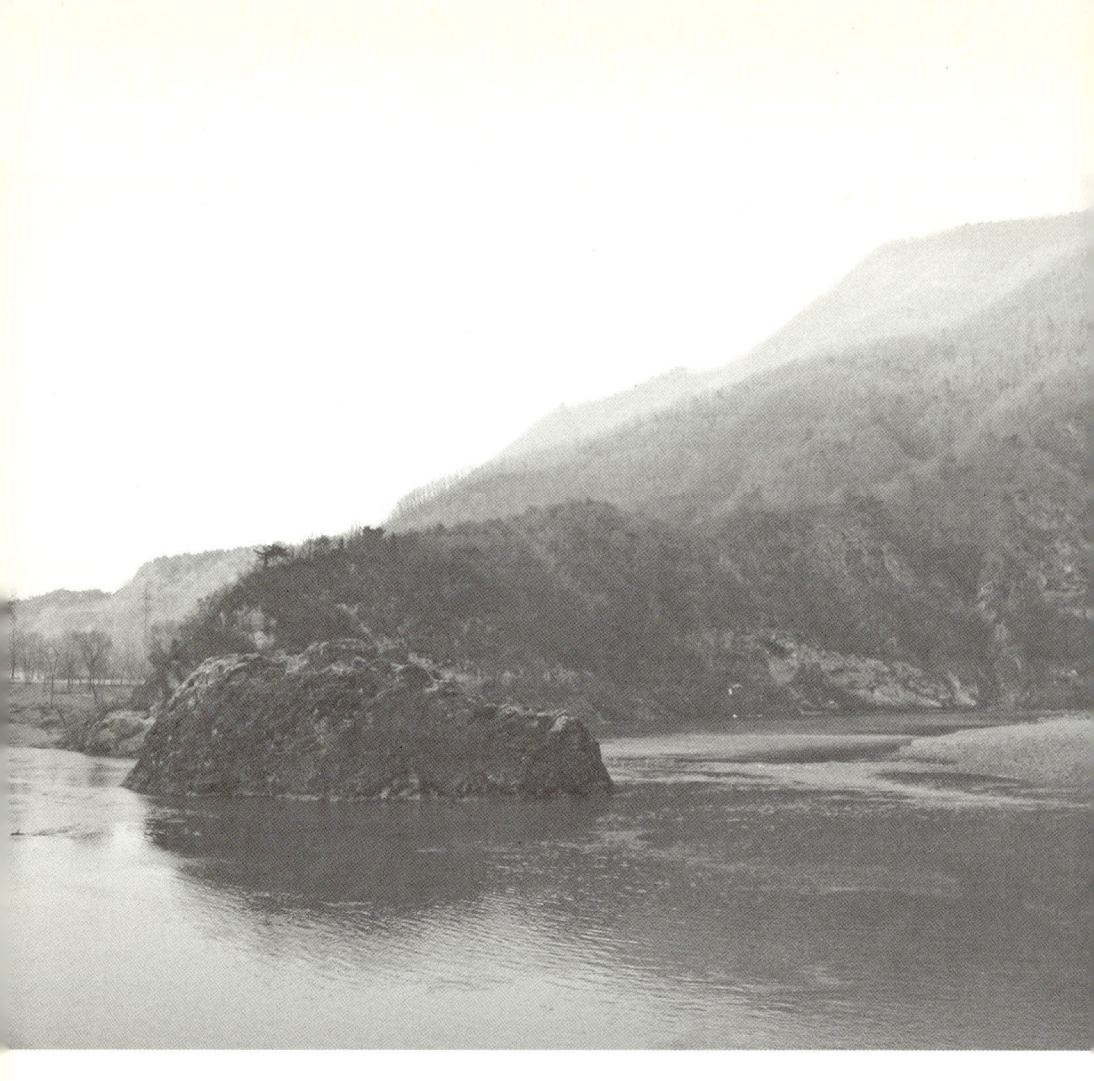

Unprepared farewell makes regret.
You should fiercely ask yourself
lest the regret just remains the regret.

The Biggest Task in My Life

Questions like where we are from before obtaining this body and where we are heading after using up this body are not only for monks up on a mountain. Mother's death is the starting point to have such a big question in my life.

A great shock came into our home which was bigger than the fact that I realized I had been a babe in the woods before coming to Seoul. My big sister who was working in the very first Korean department store as a manager announced that she would run her own business.

Since my parents were active in educating their children regardless of their gender, it would be disappointing for them that the daughter, a college graduate, did a business instead of being an educator. And soon, my big brother who was a newspaper reporter suddenly said that he would go to Germany to study. My parents decided to support their first son and daughter so they had to sell their little land and mountain back in hometown.

After that time, my family's fortune was instantly on the wane that I had to worry about my junior high tuition. My mother couldn't help but go back go hometown to collect debts from the villagers. The debt amounted to 600 thousand hwan, which is now considered some hundred million won[4]. I still remember that her back looked so forlorn when heading to hometown. It was widely said back in hometown that, I didn't know how people know that, my family had already failed so mother usually came back to Seoul with a sack of potatoes placed on her head rather than paid debts.

One day, I saw my mother weep grabbing father's hands from a crack in the door. It seemed that she was insulted with a foul tongue in hometown. Sorrow of my mother who was infinitely strong for me was a pain like my whole world crashed down. With a potato sack for which a strong man would feel too much, how difficult it would be throughout her journey from hometown

---

4) About one hundred thousand US Dollar

to Seoul by train and bus and how sorrowful she would feel. It might be why mother always said that she had a headache and she heavily depended on headache pills. What I certainly learned was that people paid their debts to successful people but not to those who were known to be a failure.

The most regretful thing of my life happened in my middle school days. One day when I was a senior, mother hurriedly left the house early in the morning for hometown. It was around the time I should leave for school and I wanted to avoid taking the same bus with mother so I deliberately waited the bus at the next stop. The bus arrived at the stop I was waiting and mother called my name and waved at me inside the bus. At that moment, I didn't take the bus but just stood still with my head bowed for a while. It was so obvious that my mother was calling my name. It was not because I hated mother. It was because my adolescent pride was hurt and I couldn't acknowledge the reality that mother couldn't help but keep going to hometown where she was not welcomed at all. After my mother passed away, this remained the most regretful in my entire life. Why couldn't I wave back smiling and wishing her a safe journey? I determined innumerably that I would never do such a mean thing in the future. Since then, unknown pent-up anger has started to be placed in my heart.

Later, we had to sell off our house in Seoul, the very last thing.

I graduated middle school in that year and I thought that even a 3000-won yearbook was extravagance so I didn't buy it. Leaving friends smiling and taking pictures with families and the yearbook behind, I got out from school in a hurry only with a diploma in my arms, not looking back even once, determining I would delete all the memories from middle school at the very moment.

I obtained a scholarship when I was a high school sophomore so I paid my tuition first and then bought gifts for my homeroom teacher and my family members. I gave my mother a handkerchief with pink embroidery and outer socks which were sold at Myeongdong Shinsegae Department Store and the money left. Mother was so happy that the baby of the family received a scholarship but she keeled over from a brain hemorrhage that year and passed away in 45 days. The last moment to see my mother was when I had no choice but to leave the hospital for finals. Since mother was paralyzed on one side, she slightly opened her one eye all the time and her big eye welled up with tears which she resisted to shed. She took me by my hand tightly and didn't let go her hold particularly on that day. All these years, I cannot ever forget how tight her grasp was. She seemed to have something she wanted to talk to me with her very last energy but she couldn't even wish me good luck for the exam. She certainly had something to tell me with holding my hands eagerly.

Unexpectedly losing my mother and arranging her keepsakes, I found the handkerchief cherished deep in a wardrobe. As if she had tried to commemorate that it was the gift from the baby, she had it with creased notes in it. I can never forget the regret I had back then. For a while, I used to habitually call "Mom" and yank the door open only to realize the room was empty, there wasn't my mother, and I couldn't see my mother ever again. The saddest thing was my despair that I couldn't do anything behind my mother's death.

Mother's death and my mental wandering after that gave me a big question on life, death and life. That was what I was wondering. Every mother and child in the world has their own story but I had to settle a problem from message that 18 years of connection with my mother left in my life. I once read a poem *Life Written at Night*[5] by Mokwol Park in high school and visited his place on Wonhyoro to ask him the meaning of loneliness and I made efforts to seek answers on life and death through exploring Buddhist philosophy and theology to ease my endless sorrow for mother's death.

---

[5] *Life Written at Night* is the essay on loneliness, eternity, life and happiness by Mokwol Park, a representative poet of Korea.

Over time, I realized that the tears shed upon mother's death were not for mother but for my sake who hadn't been ready for her death. Unprepared farewell makes regret. You should fiercely ask yourself lest the regret just remains the regret. Other than human beings, even numerous stars in the sky cannot avoid the natural laws of the huge cosmos of creation and dissipation and start and end. As even one clump of grass in a field and a small bird flying in the sky all have reasons for their being and connection for their lives, questions like where we are from before obtaining this body and where we are heading after using up this body are not only for monks up on a mountain. Mother's death is the starting point to have such a big question in my life.

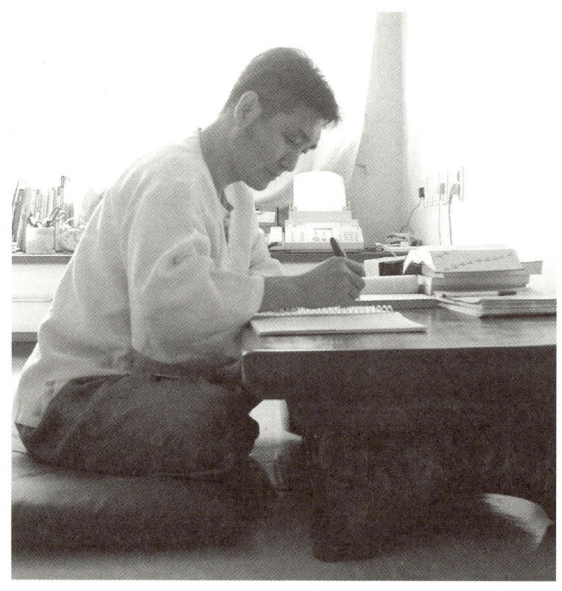

Priest, Buddhism and Connection
With determining to give back the change, I visited Dosunsa on holiday.

In the year when my mother passed away, we moved to Sungin-dong, Jongro-gu once again. I went to an institute near my house at that time during the winter vacation.

One day, I took a bus for Sinseol-dong after the institute class. After passing some blocks, a Buddhist priest got on the bus. Looking around inside the bus, the priest slowly came near where I sat. I instinctively yielded up my seat to him without knowing it. The priest smiled, thanked me and took the seat and we had a small talk.

Not long after he said he got off and would pay my bus fare instead and I didn't know why. I gave him back the change of 50 won I received from a bus conductor but he just said it was OK. I asked him where he stayed and he said it was Dosunsa temple and that was all. He got off the bus and walked away in a hurry.

Throughout the week, I couldn't get the priest out of my head. With determining to give back the change, I visited Dosunsa on holiday. Later, I came to know that the priest who paid my fare was a vice-chief priest of Dosunsa. Unfortunately, he had left for America for propagation the day before I visited. I couldn't hide my despondency. I sometimes think of what kind of relationship we would have if the connection with him lasted up to this day.

With such a small chance of encounter, I came to read a practice collection with life story of Dosunsa and Priest Cheongdam. With the collection, I found the background of Priest Cheongdam's leaving home and his humane agony in family affairs. Priest Cheongdam was a close companion of Priest Seongcheol, led a cleanup movement in Japanese-styled Buddhism in Korean[6] and worked hard for the revival of Buddhism in 1960s.

---

6) The Japanese Government-General of Choson enacted a law for the direct control of the temple management, property and monks in order to keep the Korean temple of Korea from being the base of independence movement and to damage the spirit of Korea.

Through a priest at Dosunsa, I came to know Priest Cheondam, a great Buddhist priest, and with this connection, I have become interested in Buddhism seriously.

It was never easy, however, to understand mu-sang (impermance), the core idea of Buddhism, in my late teens. Priests' expressions that everything went along connections were particularly incomprehensible for me and I sometimes felt Buddhism was like fatalism or skepticism in a way.

However, because my mother visited a temple for her entire life, I went to Jogyesa and participated in Buddhism student council for some time, expecting to get solving clues for my mother's death. No matter how hard I tried, however, I couldn't understand what priests said in a temple.

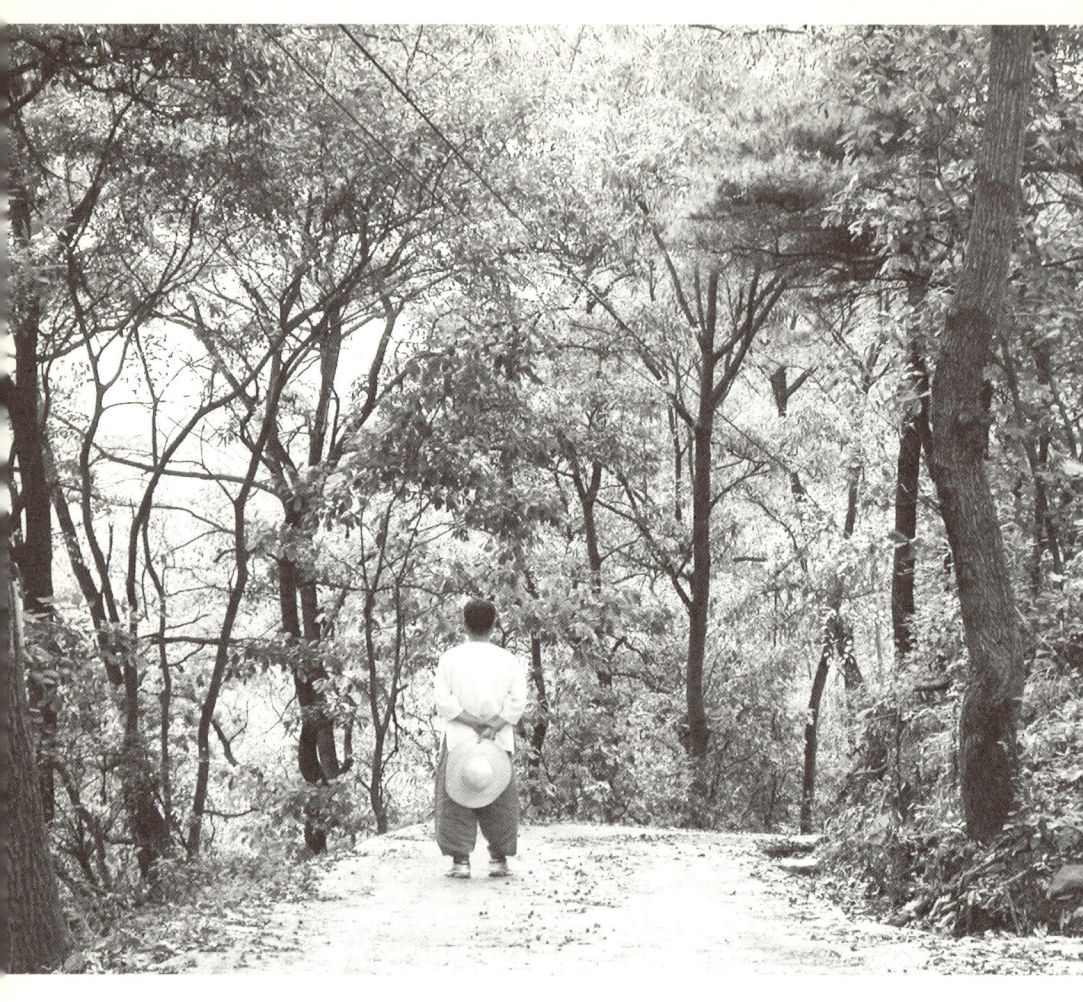

There are various ways in life.
No matter what one chooses,
the choice is upon oneself.

Four Pillars, Eight Characters and Schopenhauer

All conscious revolutions in life come in one's youth.

I got interested in sa-ju-pal-ja (four pillars and eight characters[7]) after the Buddhism. It was because what my mother said in my 3rd or 4th year at elementary school suddenly crossed my mind. Holding my hand tight and going across Dong-gang Bridge

---

7) Four pillars and eight characters is a Chinese, Japanese and Korean conceptual term that describes the four components creating a person's destiny or fate. It is called Eight Characters because each of the four pillars (representing the year, month, day, and hour of one's birth respectively) is represented by two characters.

in my hometown, she said 'You are with four pillars to be a judge or a spiritual leader. You should study hard from now on to be a great man. And you should be always honest.'

I didn't know what a judge was or pay attention to her saying when I heard that but, after her death, I came to vaguely wonder if I could really become a judge as she had said. From that day on, I started being interested in four pillars of destiny. I felt like I could figure out why my mother passed away so fast only with 18 and half years beside me if I understood it.

I didn't mean to be a fortune teller, though. It was from pure curiosity that I had an interest in oriental philosophy and four pillars of destiny. Without a concrete plan like 'I would major in this or that field,' I just studied oriental and occidental philosophies unconditionally at that time. I did have many difficulties in solving questions on death all by myself but, I was afire more fiercely in certain aspects. The way I have a critical mind or my topic started from that moment.

Four pillars of destiny is study to define myeong (Buddhist sacred wisdom for escaping from inanity and obtaining spiritual enlightenment) and reason in life with four pillars which are the year, the month, the day and the time of one's birth and eight characters among the sexagenary cycle. To foretell a person's future is now recognized just as exerting wizardry or a technique for commercial use but, from a yogic perspective, it is rather close to focused meditation. When our ancestors told fortunes before something big, they gathered a gwae (trigram from the Book of Changes), calculated the probability and took their course of that day after performing their ablutions and concentrating their mind. A War Diary describes a scene that admiral Yi Sun-shin calmed himself down and read his future before a battle. It uses a trigram from the Book of Changes only as a means but it actually requires a high level of concentration of mind for that behavior.

The question I have in studying oriental studies and four pillars of destiny is whether twins with the exactly same year, month, day and time of birth would have the same destiny if the destiny depends on the four pillars. In terms of time, 24 hours in a day are divided into twelve terrestrial branches with two hours in each and Tokyo time is used in Korea. The Tokyo time has a gap of thirty two minutes from Korean time _{which is of course reflected in four pillars of destiny}. In spite of that, it is wondered how numerous people born in the same terrestrial branch, the two hours, can have the same destiny.

My answer on this is that four pillars have more importance on time elements affecting human beings and spatial ones are excluded. Even though people are born at the same time, their backgrounds are in infinite variety. People always have regional difference like they are born in America, Africa, Jeju Island or Seoul and the environment surrounding them like parents and home background surely affects a person's future as well. In these days when parents' tremendous supporting is required to make their children go to a good university, the environment is critical in one person's life. Thus, the conclusion I drew back then was I sympathized with four pillars of destiny but it was about statistics on all human beings.

My study of life beginning in my late teens, I believe, has made my consciousness keen and delicate. I sometimes even feel as if I were seeing through a book with a hole on it. All of my fierce study, at the end, was to meet my mother. In my memory, mother was beautiful, earnest and full of convictions. While she was such a dignified amazon, she was so much heartwarming as well. Then what made her leave so early? I had to solve that question.

I had to study and earn college money at the same time. I sometimes felt dejected that I had to take responsibility for financial situations and I couldn't do what I wanted even though I had so many things I wanted to do. My only pleasure back then was books. I read some books carefully or just underlined incomprehensible ones but the books were my sole happiness and source of energy. And, though it was only ideological, I came to recognize essentials of existence in my own way.

One day in winter, I bought bagfuls of books in Jongro and happily waited an intercity bus heading for Anyang to go back home. If my memory serves me right, it cost 200 won to go from Gwancheol-dong, Jongro to Anyang. I smelled a bean-jam bun nearby, waiting for the bus. I only had 200 won for the bus after buying all those books. Because I was so cold and hungry, I finally gave up taking the bus and got the bun. So I had to walk home in Anyang from Jongro in the biting winter wind with a bag full of books on my back.

Maybe I could have talked to a bus conductor that I would take the bus for distance which my money could take me to. But, I was more inflexible than I am now and I was not the kind of guy asking things for people so I couldn't help but look for trouble myself. Looking backward, I had some kind of regret hidden in such behaviors. I tried everything to forget sorrow from losing my mother only to keep wandering because I didn't know how. I couldn't satisfy my thirstiness on things afire inside me that I wanted to know. Even with such incandescence, I somewhat tended to lean toward pessimism because I was so much fascinated with Schopenhauer. As a self-supporting student with realistic burden, that would be a matter of course. I understood Schopenhauer or Hermann Hesse only partially because I was not well established philosophically as well as translators and social atmosphere did not understand those things thoroughly.

When I encountered them again later, however, everything looked so different. For example, Schopenhauer's famous saying that 'Young men don't know how short women's beauty lasts' was just narrowly understood in my early 20s that young men and women stood for biological genders and I thought it would be unhelpful for studying to be in a relationship. So I was inclined to drive my area of activity that way.

When I came to meditate that phrase again later, however, I realized that the saying was not pessimistic but it was a metaphor from Buddhist insight. As a westerner, he was a man who was exposed to Buddhism early and opened his eyes to the concept of musang (impermanace). Young men were for youth and women's beauty was for sensuous enjoyment of youth. It would be a metaphor that it is already late if one does not have questions on existence in one's youth but travels around flowers and sucks honey from them.

Thus, wise men both of East and West say that enlightenment comes in one's youth. As people get older, they come to have more thoughts. More thoughts make energy go from abdomen to head, which erodes power of execution. Therefore, spiritual revolution in life comes in one's youth. Buddha and Jesus also reached the peak of the consciousness in their early 30s. Those who do not get afire, study or work with a determination that they would go to the end cannot ever stand on their feet in this social structure which makes our lives so dependent.

    I sometimes think that I could have had my eyes opened to life at such a young age because my home had completely collapsed. That was an experience of falling from heaven to hell. But I was dashed so fast and I had no time to recognize my suffering. I was with the determination that I had to survive in the tough life. Looking backward, I was the pain itself before I recognized it and later I became aware that it had been rather fortune.

Power of a Baked Sweet Potato

I didn't lose confidence that all the pains would mature my life directly and indirectly because that was the most valuable inheritance from my mother.

I went through a hard time physically in my 20s but I could get out of obsession with money thanks to my parents in my childhood. Maybe due to that period, I was economically deprived but I didn't feel regretful for being too much conscious of the poverty itself. What made my life difficult was rather the fact that I couldn't completely devote myself to studying with financial problems and the gloomy reality in Korea where it seemed impossible to display one's ability owing to regionalism, school relations and kinship. So, I so much wanted to go to US to study in my 20s. I wanted to test myself if it would be that hard to obtain success with the utmost efforts. To study in US, however, was way too far from the reality I was confronted with. Everyone recalls and misses their youth but it was such a hard time for me.

I recently resumed eating onions but hadn't touched them until 2004. In my early 20s, my sisters and brothers were scattered for their lives so there was a time when only I and my father lived together. We once had eaten only kimchi, onions and red pepper paste for 6 months but, when we ate up kimchi, we had no choice but to eat just on rice and onions. I had eaten numerous onions day after day but I hadn't thought that I had been in poverty. I just recalled the fact some time later that I had eaten onions for a while. That was when plain bread had just been released so I sometimes wanted to eat it when seeing people around eating the bread and drinking milk. I seldom got gluttonous over anything but I did have something I wanted to eat. Maybe because I didn't have nourishing food enough, I was all skin and bones weighing 54kg back then.

I once stayed at a reading room[8] for a while. It was somewhat

---

8) Reading room is the paid service to be used for students and ordinary people to prepare intensively to various tests. Because it is available at low fees and running for 24 hours, it is used as a housing at a low cost.

impoverished and rough days but I had a pleasant memory that I gave speeches about my immature philosophies to high school or college students younger than me who stayed up late studying in the reading room. Perhaps for that reason, they came to consult with me about their lives. Even I was uncertain about my future or career but anyway, I gave them lots of advice with Tolstoy's expressions. I cannot remember all of the advice but I vaguely remember telling them that they should define their view of life first before establishing the view on occupation. I was saying that no matter what kind of field we were in, it was required to have a belief at least in which line to take. Without that value established, we would waste our lives peeking around, not even fixing self-centeredness. I have thought this way so far and it is one of my speeches frequently given to my disciples.

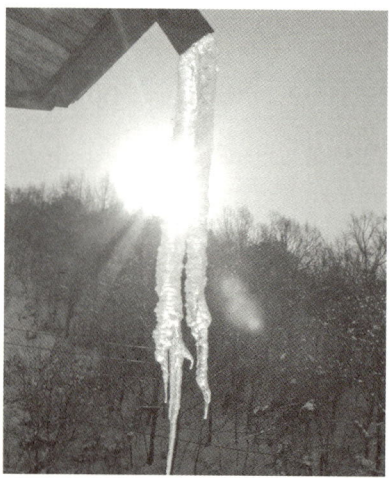

It was much colder in winter than it is now. I used to turn army blanket around myself and barely stick out my hand to turn a page. Then I could feel my warm breath on my numb fingertip. The strange feeling I had when the chill on fingertip met the breath was really something to inflame my fighting spirit. Looking back, it was maybe because of my spirit becoming stronger when things got worse. Now I think it was the study.

When students studied all night before exams, the reading room owner sometimes came in to give them a baked sweet potato and I cannot ever forget its taste. I realized that even just a piece of sweet potato had the power to change universe. It was not simply because it satisfied my hunger but it surely had the power and meaning beyond its being of food. Can I put, with my earnest energy and that of sweet potato being perfectly fit, they explosively boosted the speed of my study? I felt so much powerful as if I had a batch of it just for one potato. My pleasure from that sweet potato can be compared to the military of Goguryeo[9] that ran out of food in battlefield, received military provisions and then reaffirmed their resolve to the next battle. If I thought of reading a book to 50 pages, I determined once again to read a

---

9) Goguryeo is an ancient Korean empire flourished on a vast expanse of land in East Asia.

book through with the potato.

I could comfort myself even in sleeping on chairs put together in the reading room late at night because I had teachers like Tolstoy in my life.

I used to think, 'Tolstoy who lived a much more wealthy life than I gave his wealth and honor to the poor and left such books for people like me. And he met his death forlornly at a nameless whistle stop. So, this is nothing compared to his life. My present hardship will surely help to understand the human life comprehensively some day.'

Encouraging myself that way, I promised to regain my footing and to honorably show myself in the world. I could endure physical hunger but couldn't satisfy my fundamental hunger for essentials of life. I once demonstrated bravado while cursing heaven for the hard things given to me. But, I didn't lose confidence that absolute affirmation on me and all the pains would mature my life directly and indirectly because that was the most valuable inheritance from my mother.

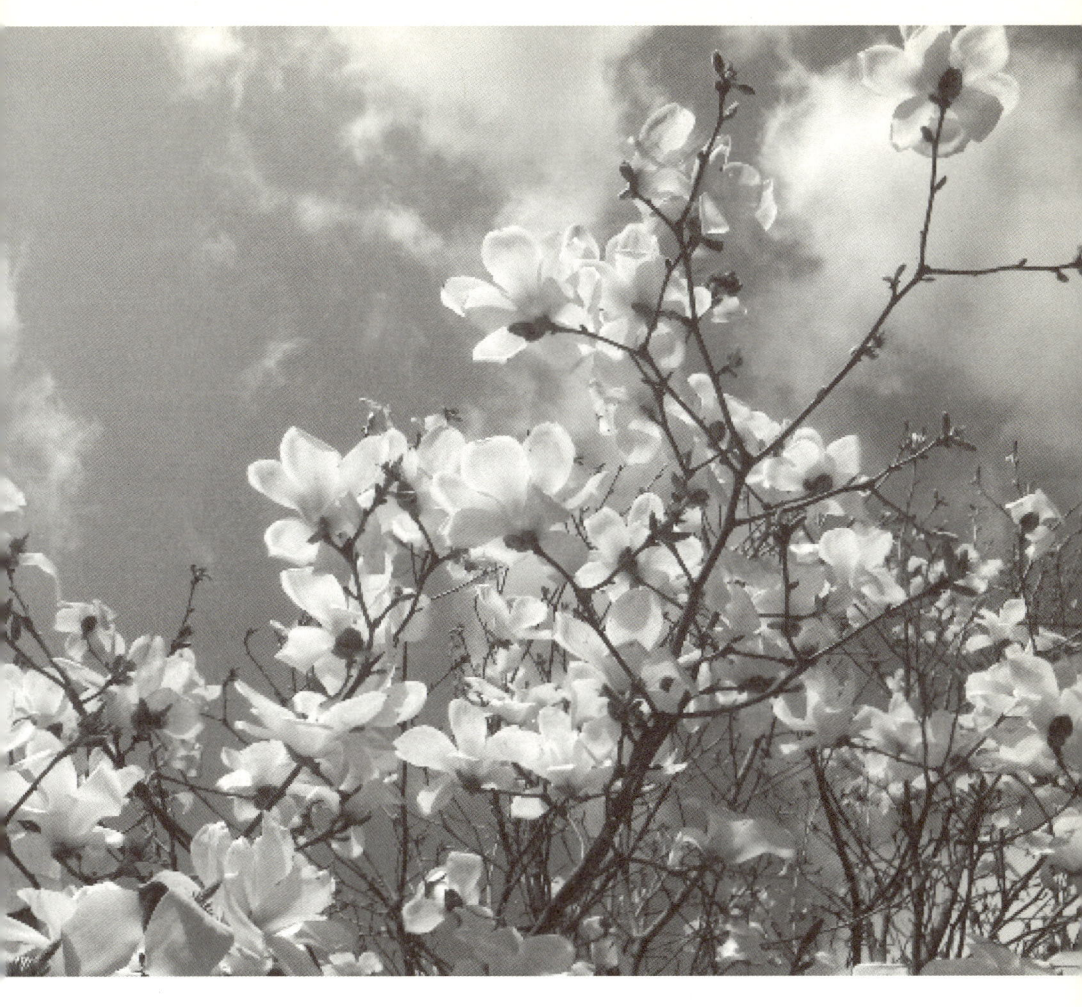

In meditation, we come to know
that hidden virtue is oddly displayed
when things are not easy but tough in life.

Mother and Udambara

What my mother left to me was faith, sincerity and the lesson
that I should never lose absolute affirmation on myself
in any difficult circumstances.

It has been thirty years in 2005 since my mother died. Yes. It's been thirty years, the one generation. If it had not been for my mother, I couldn't walk along this way until this moment when I study yoga. Looking back to the track of the time, I am sure that what has made me to be here is not only my efforts. I have always had people supporting me whenever I met hard situations and I have also felt that hidden virtue of my parents was subtly there when I was at crossroads for making important decisions.

This year, Udambara bloomed at Jongro branch and it became an issue. Udambara, the legendary flower, is known as numinous flower frequently appearing in many Buddhist scriptures so people say it is an auspicious sign for it to catch people's eye. It is Jogyesa which is across from Jongro institute where we commemorated 49th day after mother's death and the day I was told Udambara bloomed was when the 49th day after mother's death was finished thirty years ago. There has been scientific controversy over authenticity of Udambara but it wouldn't be a mere coincidence that I immediately recalled my mother at the very moment when I heard of it. She was a sincere Buddhist and I remember an anecdote related to her mind as a Buddhist.

It has probably been more than forty years. Mother went to a temple in hometown the day before Buddha's birthday. She and other Buddhists staying together decided to put up lotus lanterns at dawn on Buddha's birthday and went to bed. My mother, however, was in a deep sleep so it was already late when she went out to hang lanterns. She saw that all the good places had been already taken and only edges were left. The edges were where wind was the most directly blowing so everyone else avoided. She couldn't help but hung lanterns there and they seemed shaky with wind as expected. Thinking for a while, she picked up some pebbles and put them at both ends of lanterns so that lanterns got balanced and shook less with the weight and then she returned to the room. After the day broke, people were gathered around the eaves where lanterns were hung so my mother went there to see what had happened. What people were looking at was the mother's lanterns burning to the last without wavering because other lanterns were blown out for wind and rain at daybreak.

Telling me that story from time to time, my mother said numerous times that Buddha's energy was with us if we had sincerity and faith. When I went to temples with mother in my childhood holding her hands, I was always told 'You will succeed. So you should live with confidence and belief in yourself.' What my mother left to me was faith, sincerity and the lesson that I should never lose absolute affirmation on myself in any difficult circumstances. It is these three that I always emphasize to disciples at the institute.

We should not ever give up meditative life no matter how hard our lives can get and, in meditation, we come to know that hidden virtue is oddly displayed when things are not easy but tough in life. The power invisible in a faint hope at a decisive and desperate moment! You will find out the hidden virtue is working.

Bongsun Sitting with Vajrasana

Master, no matter how hard it is,
do not be upset and have a gentle mind. It is good to be nice.

It has been nearly ten years to build this training institute and to be settled here in Dongnyang-myeon, Chungju-si. People who make their first visit here wonder how I came to find this beautiful place and how I obtained it as one. Actually, I can just say this ground and I should have a connection.

Two to three years before coming here, I had gone around from suburbs of Seoul to the whole area of Gyeonggi-do, Gangwon-do and Chungcheongnam-do and Chungcheongbuk-do to search for proper place for training institute on holidays or whenever I had free time. I visited several places but ones I loved had already been taken with the rich people's villas or training institutes of businesses and others which were not bad were breathtaking expensive that I couldn't even bring it up. Sometimes I found sites I liked with good price. They were good at the first sight but they looked like a grave lot on my way back. It didn't seem easy to carry out my plans to leave a complex city and to finish my studying in such a neat training institute when I got older.

Looking back what I planned and pushed ahead, I came to think whether this project had something inconsistent or wrong. A few days after having this thought, I dreamed a dream. Because I seldom had dreams, I thought carefully about it. I drew a conclusion the dream meant that graves of my parents which had been separate from each other should be together and because my mother passed away earlier, I set the date to move the mother's grave to where my father lied down. Soon after moving my mother, I dreamed once more and I came to find this ground and have been settled to the present. People talk about dreams a lot like they win the lottery or pass a big exam after having a dream with dragon or pig in it. I think the dreams I had back then were fundamentally different from those kinds of dreams.

According to what villagers said, this ground used to be called tiger valley (Beom-gol) because there had been tigers around here. I thought it was likely that way in the past because even most villagers felt this ground was deep in mountains in spite of the fact that the place was just 700 or 800 meters away from the village. Hearing what they said, I renamed the place phoenix valley (Bong-gol) myself as it would be auspicious ground where many people would come to study health and wisdom from that time on. Since then, villagers as well as teachers have called the place phoenix valley.

For the first six month in this backwoods, I was with a brace of little Poongsan dogs. The male was named Baw because my hometown Gangwon-do was called 'Potato Baw' which meant a potato farmer in Korean. The female was called Bongsun combining Bong of Bong-gol and Sun (which was one of the most commonly used girls' names in Korea). Three of us – I, Baw and Bongsun – had lived in this backwoods for six months with no one else. I looked after the two puppies back then instead they guarded me.

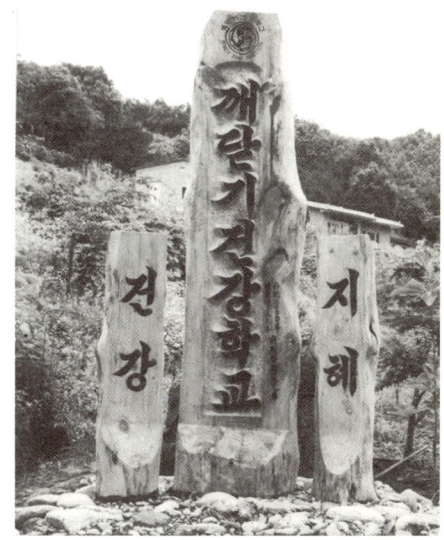

The institute was called Health Enlightenment School to open up enlightenment in health and wisdom in its early days.

Mother, My Lifelong Topic

Bongsun was just a month old when she came here and I decided to make her the bride of six-month-old Baw. She was all white and as small as palm so people who see Bongsun after she has all grown up cannot even imagine what she was like back then. Now, Bongsun is like an unpopular, plump lady for a person.

Bongsun used to whine and cry and bark at or fight against Baw that was three or four times bigger than her but she stopped barking after she began growing out of a puppy. One-year-old dogs are an adult for human being but she didn't bark even when she was almost two. It is natural for dogs to bark at strangers but she never did it so I was wondering if she forgot how to bark or she didn't know it from the beginning. I was also worried if something was wrong with her. One summer day in 1999, all of a sudden, she barked for the first time, which was such a resonant bark reminding me of the roar of a tiger or a lion. The bark as powerful as Baw's made the entire Bong-gol resonated. How delighted and amazed I was···

In spite of that, one of the Bongsun's biggest characteristics is she hardly barks at strangers compared to Baw, Sundol – her young – and Jinsun, a Jindo dog[10] living with us here. Bongsun

---

10) Jindo Dog is National Treasure of Korea and well known for their high intelligence, loyalty, fighting spirit and its beautiful appearance.

barks in two cases only and one is when a strange man appears in the territory she feels responsible for. She never barked even when hundreds of women walked around her. We concluded that she would think 'Oh, our members are here today to practice. Why does Jinsun keep barking at them? It so gets in the way of their studying.' She didn't bark at a strange man until he came in her territory. Having faith in roles of Baw, Sundol and Jinsun, she never overstepped their authority. So we thought she was really smart. She also barks while staring at a distant mountain with full moon constantly over an hour. She may practice mantra[11] with valor devotion once a month.

Bongsun in Bong-gol is not particular about foods so one virtue of hers is to eat all her meal and leave nothing. Her bowl looks as if it were washed up because she licks up the bowl like Buddhist priests have their meal, which is known as leaving nothing behind and called Balwu-gongyang in Korean. And she sometimes belches like humans. When she leaves food or skips meals occasionally, it means she is particularly sick. She eats anything

---

11) It means 'thoughts or intention expressed with sound' and it is translated into recitation, the words of Buddha, prayer, advice, plan, etc. Mantra is a numinous and supernatural phoneme and Aum, a representative mantra, is a holy sound including start–process–end of universe or birth–life–death. Mantra yoga is a branch of orthodox yoga.

even grass. Dogs are omnivores but they are originally carnivorous so it is unusual for her to eat grass. She does so because, for example, she takes it as a medicinal herb she needs.

Bongsun likes fruits, vegetables, grass and kimchi so much. Throughout all spring and summer, Bongsun takes yellow dandelions when she gets bored, throws away its leaves and digs up the root with her front paws and eats it. She also likes mugwort a lot so we would say she will be a human soon only if she eats garlic while seeing her eat the mugwort with relish. In summer, she is so enthusiastic over watermelons – her favorite, – corns, potatoes, cabbages, tomatoes, plums and cucumbers and, in fall, sweet potatoes, napa cabbages and apples. She puts apples or corns between her front paws and gnaws upon them with front teeth. She also enjoys dried sea tangle and even chili. One day, when I was picking chili from our field and planning to dry them in the sun, she wagged her tail around me. I was not sure but gave her some and she ate them away, smacking her lips to ask for more. She seems depressed if she

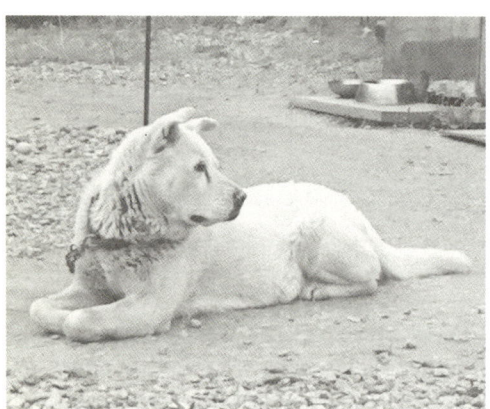
Our Bongsun sitting with vajrasana!

hasn't eaten fresh fruits and vegetables for a while, so people would say something like they don't know whether Bongsun is a dog or a cow.

Though no one has taught her, Bongsun in Bong-gol has a habit of sitting on her front legs with vajrasana which is of sitting on one's knees. She seems to meditate when sitting nonchalantly sometimes for ten or twenty minutes while looking at ridges around evening. No. Seeing her sitting that way, we would say 'Bongsun is meditating.' Coming as the institute keeper, she does not know how to bark at strangers but she wags not only her tail but her waist. Bongsun that likes everyone and that leaves no food with any complaints like Buddhist monks! It was four or five years ago when she was diagnosed with dog heartworm. Medicines for the heartworm were too strong but we gave her medicines and injections while taking risks. We were told that she might suffer from aftereffects but she has endured them well and lived bravely.

In the last sweltering summer with so much rain, however, she got ill from the heat and started to suffer from a drawn-out illness. She couldn't even walk like an old woman. We made her a patient's room and connected wires to put two fans to save her from the heat in such weather with irregular changes. All teachers at the institute looked after her over a month by turns. She would be lost in meditation singularly with hearing 'gwan-se-um bo-sal (the Buddhist Goddess of Mercy)' so the recorder was turned on all the time and she listened to it. Bongsun eventually couldn't walk so institute teachers took care of her wastes and nursed her devotedly in turn.

Bongsun, however, left us in one month and five days. We cleaned and shrouded her like people did for the dead and made a casket. We cremated her by requesting a business specialized in animal cremation and sprinkled over the mountain by the institute. We had unseasonable rain in September on the day we scattered her bones as if she had been sorry for leaving. Coming to this institute in one month after being born and living for ten y ears with her husband and child, she left this world in her base, the hometown, after being looked after more devotedly than some people at the last phase of her life. What makes me think that she would certainly be born as a great disciplinant if she were reincarnated? It has been over one month since she left but Bongsun still gives me strong impressions with her usual face and I hear her voice even in silence.

"Master, no matter how hard it is, do not be upset and have a gentle mind. It is good to be nice."
How can a dog be so docile? Throughout my life, I've never

seen any creature including humans or dogs with such gentle nature as Bongsun. It may be my first and the last to encounter that kind of gentle creature. How could Bongsun in Bong-gol be so mild and nice? Her mildness and niceness is like going toward a new hill over life's ordeal. Nonviolence of Mahatma Gandhi, one of the most respectful figures in 20th century, is ahimsa, the very first precept of ethical lesson in yoga. The more I think of memories with Bongsun, the deeper I come to meditate ahimsa.

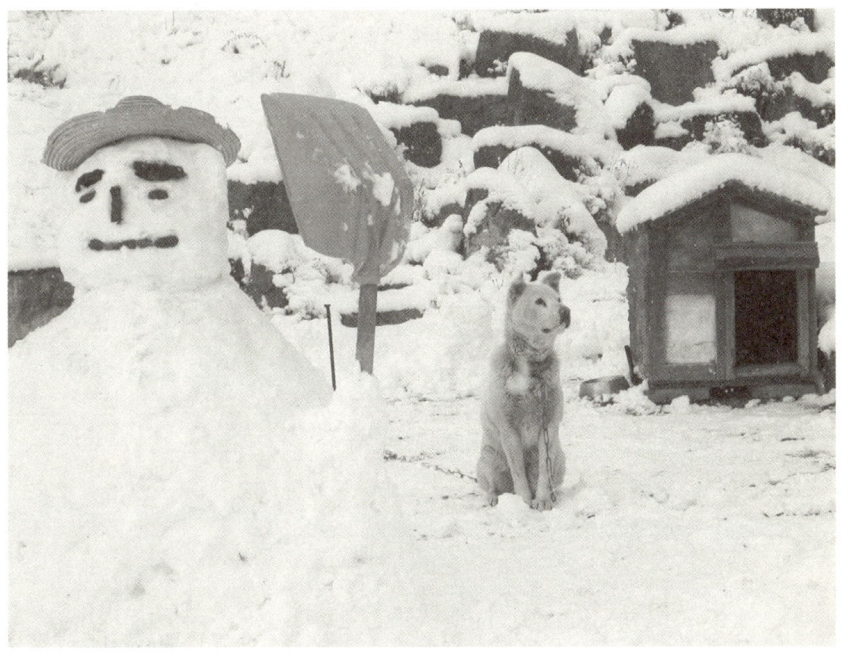

Bongsun in Bong-gol left us after living such a good life. Though she left even before she had used the solid, newly made wooden house, she would be ever alive as the gentle Bongsun in many people's hearts. Good bye, Bongsun. I hope you to be reborn as a disciplinant so that you could show many people your niceness and gentleness. Bongsun reminds me of our ancestors' old saying. 'Human beings shouldn't be inferior to dogs.' Are people inferior to dogs increasing or decreasing? The answer would be in our minds.

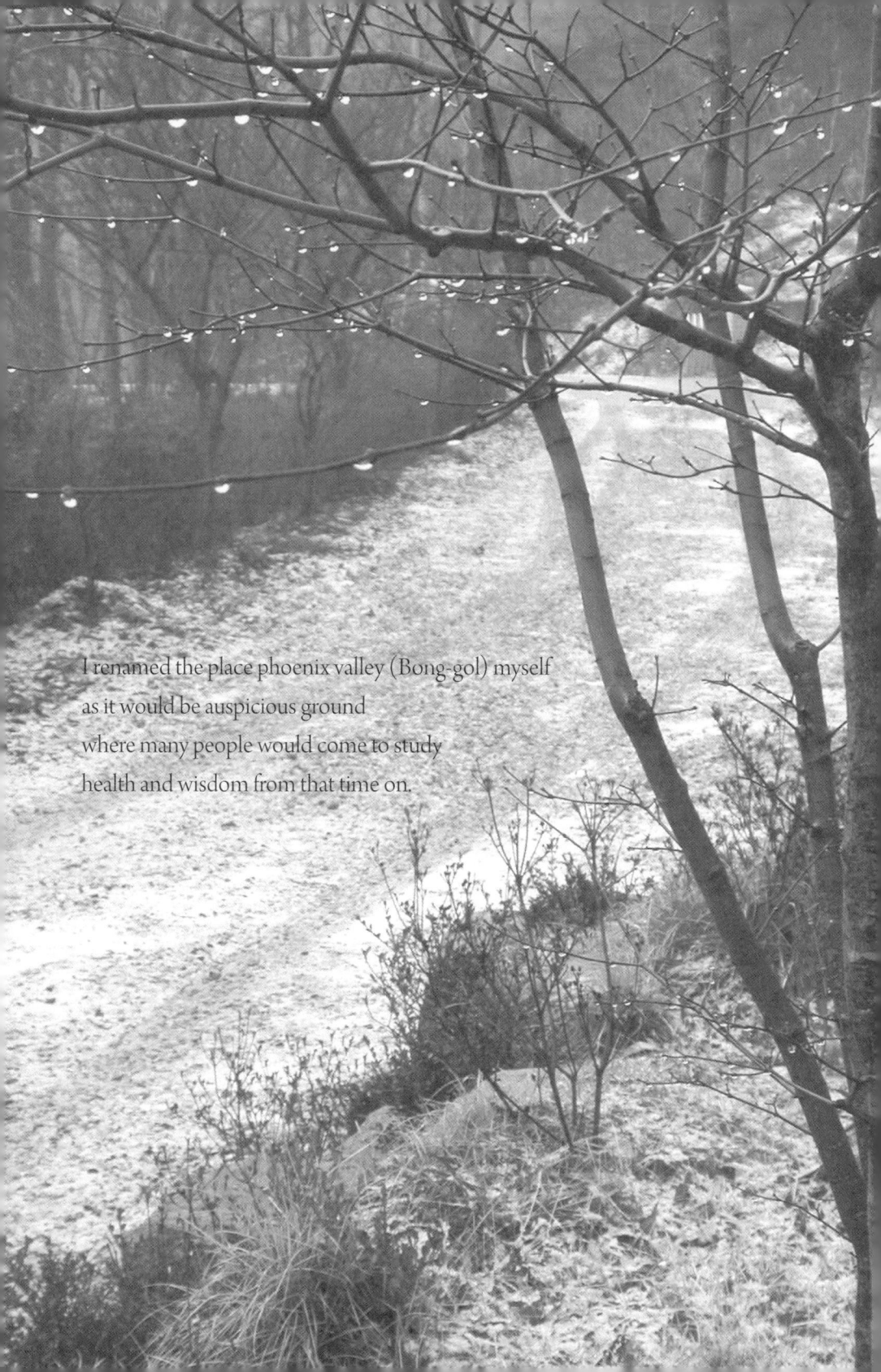

I renamed the place phoenix valley (Bong-gol) myself
as it would be auspicious ground
where many people would come to study
health and wisdom from that time on.

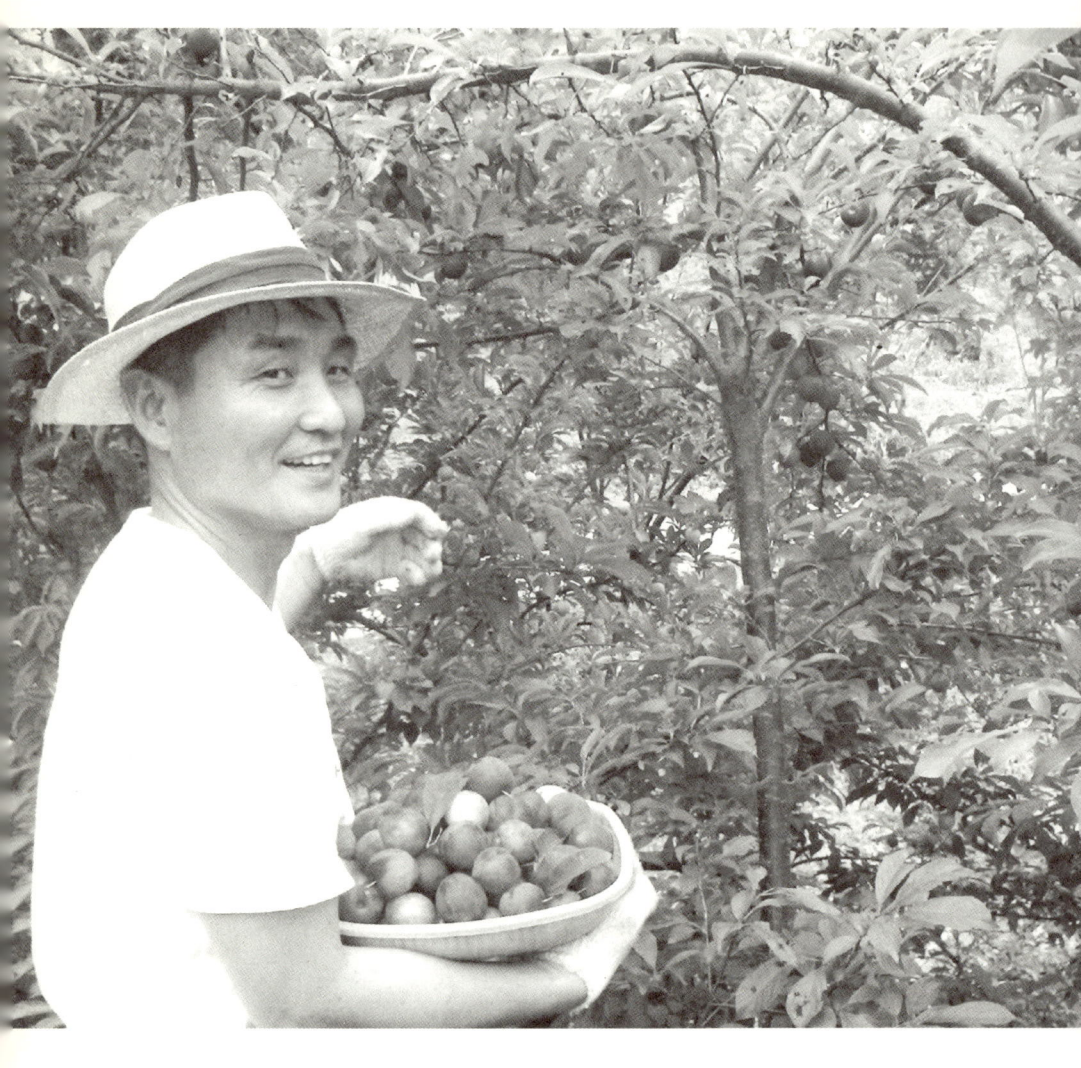

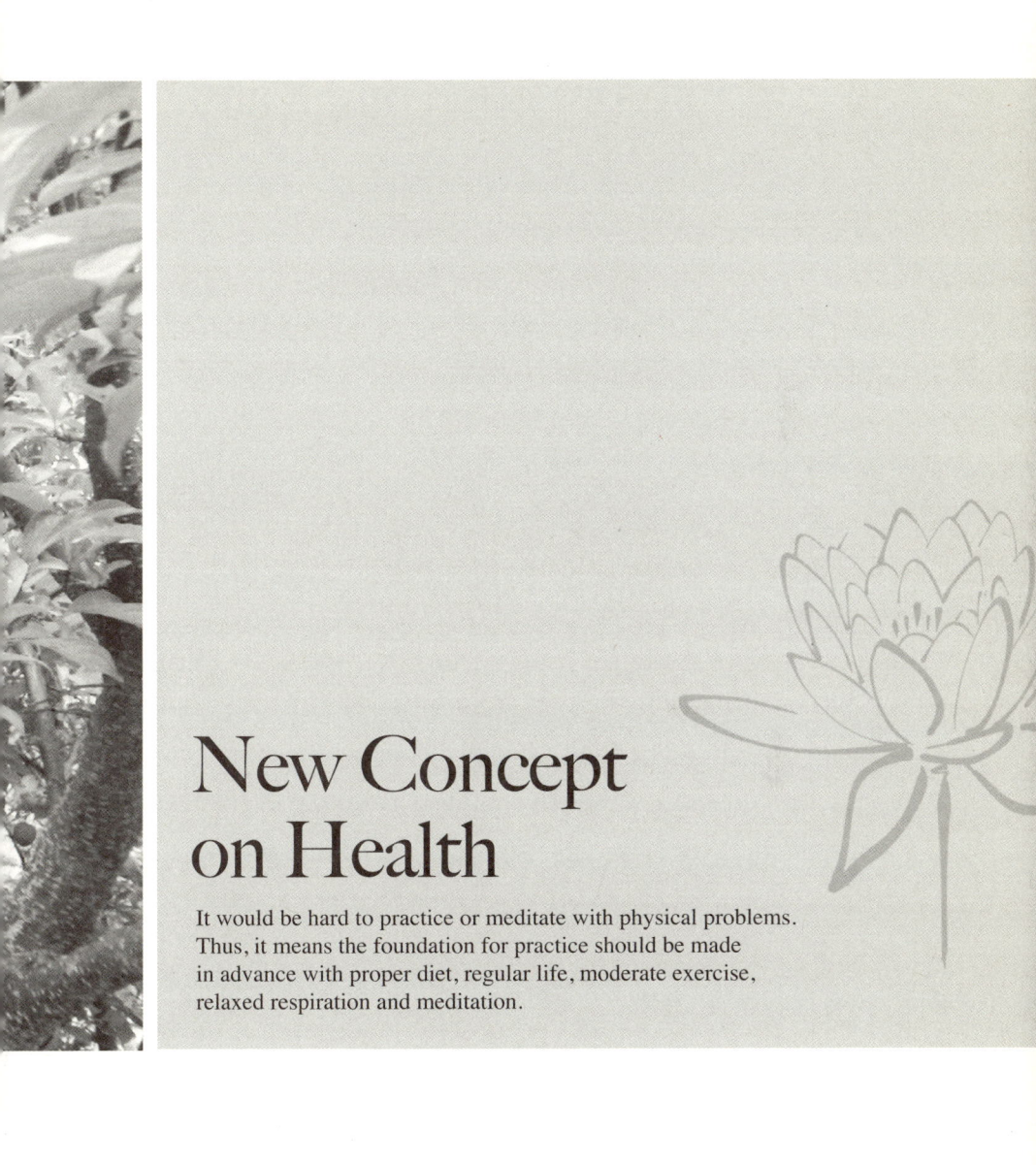

New Concept on Health

It would be hard to practice or meditate with physical problems.
Thus, it means the foundation for practice should be made
in advance with proper diet, regular life, moderate exercise,
relaxed respiration and meditation.

Reinterpretation on Health

The thing on which energy, an oriental concept, and a spiritual one are added to traditional concept of health can be an example.

People are practicing yoga in studios[12] to be healthy but most of them lack accurate recognition on health actually. People study into diseases these days, mainly thinking of how to overcome them. So, massive man power, capital and technology are input to develop new vaccines and medications worldwide each year.

---

12) Where people do yoga is not a place to learn techniques or skills but to improve their body and mind so it is called a studio.

On the other hand, they seldom think of how to be healthy. They bring the concept of health only to research some diseases. When people pay just 1% of time and efforts that are used for disease research to being healthy, there will surely be conscious changes on health. Honestly, our lives would be very tight only to think about how to be healthy. It gets simple when we concern about being healthy.

It gets complicated, however, when thinking how to treat diseases. According to WHO, there are 1.3 million kinds of illnesses analyzed so how can we memorize all of them? From a perspective of people who grasp the principles, it is considered silly to choose a challenging way over an easy one.

Health naturally comes into our lives when we have positive thinking on ourselves and we lead regular lives. It seems that the idea that all diseases should be cured is due to wrong conception on illnesses. Being healthy doesn't mean never getting ill. For example, if you catch a cold and you recover from it without the cold worsening to pneumonia, it could lower the probability of catching pneumonia with the immune system improved against colds and pneumonia. It is the same for hepatitis. Once you get immune against it, you don't have to get a vaccine. We should positively understand that illnesses can be a seed and foundation for greater health in some cases.

When we catch a disease and it naturally heals, we can be rather healthier with better immunity. Medicinal herbs in oriental medicine are extracts in general and medicinal properties of the herbs, from herbs' perspectives, are usually toxicity to protect them. Thus, toxicity becomes medication and vice versa on some occasions like bad company can sometimes be of help in life. If we see a bad guy and we can determine 'not to live like that bad guy,' we can let his bad behaviors be a good lesson to ourselves for positive life. In thinking structure of Oriental studies, being good and bad are not extremely divided and they are recognized as one and as two at the same time upon thorough understanding on their meanings.

All kinds of leaders in the past no matter what they were called such as a tribal chief or a headman were priests beyond simply being a political leader. Priests meant not only executors for sacrifices but a leader understanding principles of nature and all creation. So they were easily able to rule the subjects based on their wisdom in life without using physical strength or military force. They were also able to cure diseases by using knowledge obtained through their experience and principles they understood. Drugs are socially regulated strictly these days but there were no such concepts in the past. Drugs were not meant to be drugs but they become narcotics with people's excessive use. Therefore, any good medicines can be drugs when they are heavily used. On the other hand, medicinal herbs or grass we call drugs can be medicines according to circumstances when they are used with adequate amount upon symptoms which they act on. Today, however, people do not have accurate knowledge or wisdom for taking only by that adequate amount so it becomes impossible in reality. In old times, group leaders like a headman or a tribal chief guided their people. They knew exactly how much amount was effective based on their previous experiences. Not only did they prescribe medications but they added formality with proper rites. Through the formality, the medications were of spiritual meaning which included healing in mind as well as physical material.

Those leaders had wisdom to understand and to practice principles of nature. So the dichotomous thinking on body and mind in the West like 'diseases for doctors and spirits for catholic priests or ministers' is naturally different a lot from the oriental thinking structure. While occidental medicine has defined health as maintaining physical immunity and homeostasis, oriental medicine has considered health as harmonizing the invisible energy and visible meridian which are relative concepts of Yin and Yang to keep our bodies. In 21st century, however, the West does not limitedly regard the concept of health as a material or physical concept any more. On the existing views that being healthy is a physical, mental and social well-being without illnesses, the thing on which energy, an oriental concept, and a spiritual one are added to traditional concept of health can be an example.

Through modern scientific analyses, westerners have found that principles of acupuncture and moxibustion, the basics of oriental medicine and energy concepts related to nadis[13] in yoga are exquisitely linked to conclusions of occidental medicine so they come to embrace principles in oriental philosophies as alternative medicines which can encompass separately segmentalized studies as one big principle such as Yin-Yang Five Elements and I Ching. In other words, there are certain fundamental principles beyond perception by five senses[14] in thinking of being healthy and even Westerners have started acknowledging its actual impact on humans. Therefore, this changing culture of health should be seen with a broader view with conversion of awareness also in Korea. It is of absolute need for awareness conversion toward health.

---

13) It is a plural form of nadi. Nadi means a passage, duct or channel and it is the passage through which prana, the vitality in yoga, circulates. It is a form of interlinked energy flowing through and a concept similar to humors and pulse or meridian system in oriental medicine.
14) Five sensory organs; eye, nose, mouth, ear and skin. People receive information outside through them.

Sources for Human Food are on Heaven and Earth

Foods have their source on heaven and earth.

The sources of humans' breathing and foods are on heaven and earth. After we breathe, drink water and eat foods, we cannot gain nutrients and energies to maintain our lives without the five viscera and the six entrails' process of digestion, absorption, storage and excretion. Therefore, energy, the source of vitality, is obtained only after production progress of the five viscera and the six entrails and our nature such as health, temperament, character and tendency is subject to characteristics of the five viscera and the six entrails.

However, everyone has different innate sizes or energies in their five viscera and the six entrails and the gaps between them grow bigger based on each one's unique lifestyle or eating habit. We call it constitution that every individual comes to have in their realistic gap in energies.

The constitution in yoga is determined by combination of the three dosha; vata, pitta and kapha which mean technical principles in the body or biological power or temperament and by balance of power. Vata means wind and air and this temperament is with characteristics of dryness, coldness and mobility affecting functions like blood circulation, delivery of neural stimulation and excretion, etc. Pitta means bile and temperament with strong hotness, liquid and acridity in the body so it functions as providing heat to body and making blood get red. Kapha means phlegm and it is of heavy, cold, oily and sweet features. Depending on which temperament is dominant among the three dosha, yoga classifies constitution into three of vata, pitta and kapha.

Oriental medicine considers that health care should vary according to one's constitution. In terms of this constitution, being healthy is to get well balanced by supplementing bias of the five viscera and the six entrails and imbalance in temperament and then the constitution will also be able to be overcome.

Assuming that the five viscera and the six entrails are factories working for maintenance of our bodies, all the factories cannot realistically do the same amount of work. In some factories with less work, workers can leave at the regular time while those who in other factories with much work cannot avoid working overtime and even overnight for tight working schedule. Among those busy factories, some operate smoothly while others strike based on conditions such as their wage, working conditions, welfare benefits, labor relations and achievement, etc.

As employers' mind, management philosophy and labor relations matter in business administration, we, the master of the five viscera and the six entrails, also need certain management philosophy to rule our body. With this regard, principles of Yin-Yang and Five Elements can be a kind of management philosophy necessary to control our body. To make the five viscera and the six entrails stay healthy, balance of power should also be maintained. Each of the five viscera and the six entrails corresponding to five Elements; *mok* (wood), *hwa* (fire), *to* (earth), *keum* (iron) and *su* (water), is subject to relationship of coexistence to one-sidedly help each other, that of incompatibility to oppress energies unilaterally and that of reversed winning to hold incompatibility so the five viscera and the six entrails get harmonized and balanced by the dynamics of the three. We call it to be healthy when this balance is maintained, but otherwise we don't.

The five viscera and the six entrails are linked with other organs in the body through the energy circulation system so they mutually affect. This is called nadis on yoga and humors and pulse in oriental medicine, which can be understood as a passage through which energy interlinked in both body and mind. For example, when energy in the liver and the bowels goes wrong, other organs related to the liver and the bowels such as eye, throat, muscles, hip joint and nails can have problems. Oriental medicine, therefore, observes symptoms in the body and figures out to which organs these symptoms are involved and where they come from to prescribe medication to support those organs.

This is applied to problems in mind or mental symptoms as well as bodily ones. Modern medicine tends to analyze psychological symptoms related to various human feelings only by brains but oriental medicine regards that *o-yok-chil-jung* (humans' five desires and the seven passions) come out of the five viscera and the six entrails. Not only are physical characteristics displayed with symptoms but also problems occurring due to failure to control emotions are physical and mental disconcertion caused actually by the off-balance five viscera and the six entrails. In other words, even though our health and even emotions, thinking and will which used to be recognized as areas of one's head are output from our heads, the real source of energy that the brain uses is that very factory, five viscera and the six entrails. Some people express it as energy of the fundamental root.

Then, what makes the energy of five viscera and the six entrails? The answer is the aforementioned water, air and soil – the energy of heaven and earth – and food like grains, vegetables and fruits grown out of them from the nature. From this viewpoint, we can understand that all energies forming us are ultimately from the universe and the nature. Therefore, meditation is not the only answer to cure bodily or mental illnesses but many problems great and small can be solved in natural methods through using foods which can directly affect the five viscera and the six entrails. Here is the explanation from applying principles of Five Elements in realistic daily lives.

• Phenomenon by Five Elements •
1. Do not snack before meals

The energy of wood is one for start and development, which is the energy of spring. Recall the process of sprout's pushing the frozen ground and growing up. Compared to human body, it is the energy coming out of the liver and bowels and gall bladder and it corresponds to sour taste. People with healthy wood energy have gentle tendency, literary features and planning quality and they well display administrative ability. But when people get the wood energy excessively, however, they become incompatible with earth energy subject to spleen and stomach.

I think your parents would have told you not to snack before meals. Taking much sweets actually make people lose their appetite. That means a little salty and sour foods can put an edge on children with no appetite. Traditionally, we Koreans would have rice porridge with soy sauce on which a few drops of sesame or perilla oil are added. The salty taste of soy sauce is water energy and aromatic taste of sesame or perilla oil is wood energy as of the sour taste. These two energies oppress the earth energy according to principles of Five Elements.

Taking too much food with this wood energy goes against earth energy and this can cause problems in the stomach. In addition, greasy bread aggravates fatigue in stomach so the wall of stomach can hurt or heartburn can be developed as well. When energy in spleen and stomach gets down, people become lazy and come to have too many thoughts. It is of no use to tell them to meditate to stop thinking instead of thinking too much. The phenomenon people have many thoughts and suspicions and become lazy is because of excessive energy in the liver and bowels and gall bladder, which is incompatible with spleen and stomach. In this case, it is more realistic to give them pumpkins or honey with natural sweetness. The earth energy is stabilized by eating sweet food for better nutrition and by doing yoga postures to help spleen and stomach.

2. The reason why modern people easily get hwa-byung[15]

The fire energy is energy in summer and one for growth and development. Applying it to human body, it is energy in heart and small intestine and bitter taste among natural flavors.

In summer, heart and small intestine in our body, the organs subject to fire energy, are affected the most. So we get more stressful and annoyed in summer than any other season. People sweating a lot not even in hot summer, getting easily upset with their faces turning red or feeling their shoulders heavy and often being out of breath have these phenomena because of weak energy in heart and small intestine. Thus, they need to get balanced in their body with foods and exercise helpful for heart.

It is said that modern people generally have *hwa-byung* a lot and this *hwa-byung* literally means problems in heart, the organ with fire energy. *Byung* means an illness in Korean. It is particularly related to food culture and constitution. Koreans' foods are mainly based on soy sauce, soybean paste and red pepper paste

---

15) Hwa-Byung translates into English as anger or fire disease. It is listed in the Diagnostic and Statistical Manual, Korea Edition (DSM-K), as a typical mental illness that is found in people of Korean descent, that can make someone suddenly unable to suppress his/her emotions of anger, sadness, hurt, guilt or shame, etc for a short time, it is sometimes accompanied by incontinence (urine and/or feces).

and various kinds of kimchi which contains a lot of green onion, garlic and powered red pepper. These foods are characterized that they are subject to iron and water energy among Five Elements. The water energy in Five Elements has a feature to press heart and small intestine with fire energy. So Koreans have endurance and patience with water energy and desire for winning and leadership with iron energy but have relatively weak heart in general based on constitution.

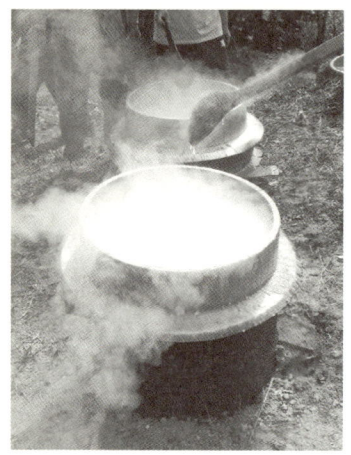
Soybeans being boiled for making fermented soybean lump

Modern people, therefore, are more likely to get *hwa-byung*. People with hwa-byung should eat foods like sorghum which tastes bitter to stabilize energy in heart. If your husband easily gets sharp temper or your children are ill-mannered and make a lot of troubles, steadily give them rice with sorghum. Over time, you can see them gradually changing.

Taking bitter food with fire energy too much, however, goes against the iron energy and this can cause lungs and large intestine to be weak. People with weak lungs and large intestine can become too negative or pessimistic. They can sometimes suffer a loss from helping others because of being too much emotional and interfering in others' businesses with excessive sympathy.

3. When having too much appetite

The earth energy is the energy of midsummer and this time of the year is mainly when we can swim. This earth energy is for maturing, changing and harmonizing. It is the same principle as a plant blooms at its peak. Applying it to human body, it is energy in spleen and stomach and sweet taste among natural flavors. People with healthy earth energy tend to do everything accurately, live with others in harmony and have firm inclination.

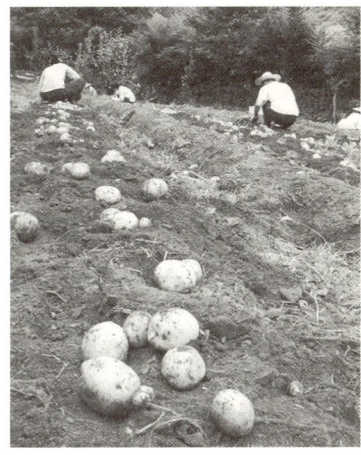

Potato harvest in international meditation Center Nae-aneui Ddeul

People say that child obesity is on the rise. To eat much is hard on a body with the work on five viscera and the six entrails aggravated and it also causes complex thinking so both mind and body can deteriorate. It is of no use to tell those who are addicted to eating not to be greedy for foods. The way is very simple. Pumpkins or honey which has natural sweetness are helpful to lower the appetite. Natural sweetness gradually lowers the level of appetite and eventually leads one to eat less. It isn't needed to keep eating pumpkins or honey and it is okay to stop when the appetite is appropriately controlled. With the diet supplementing sweetness, weight would be under control and the body get balanced little

New Concept on Health

by little while getting fresh air and taking a walk from time to time.

The earth energy among Five Elements is at the center of all energies. The center is required to take directions of north, south, east and west. Without the center, everything gets lost. Thus, people lacking the earth energy talk a lot because they feel empty inside. Talking unnecessarily too much, therefore, means having no center.

4. Spicy food is more delicious in the evening.

The iron energy is the energy of fall and it is for convergence and shrinkage. Imagine leaves falling in fall and fruits bearing in return. Applying it to human body, it is energy in lungs and large intestine and hot taste among natural flavors. People with healthy iron energy keep regular hours and have leadership and strong desire for winning.

Not many people want hot fish stew or kimchi stew for their breakfast. Hot and spicy foods appeal to people's taste when it gets chilly and cool in the evenings. The Korean food Tteokbokki, rice cakes in hot sauce, is more delicious in the evenings than in the mornings. Young people have interests in dieting increasingly, which is enough to be a social issue. To lose weight, eat spicy food. Thus, chili pepper diet was once an issue a while ago. Grilled garlic or kimchi stew with much chili powder makes people keep puffing and breathe out much. It is because the spicy taste generates heat in the body and burns body fat. The spicy taste is not only in foods like red pepper taste but in brown rice among grains. If people with weak lungs or large intestine cannot eat spicy taste, it is helpful to steadily have brown rice.

5. When our bodies lack water

The water energy is the energy of winter and it is original life energy for storage and concealment. Imagine a winter tree with bare branches and winter buds inside to get prepared for lives in spring. Applying it to human body, it is energy in kidney and bladder and salty taste among natural flavors. People with healthy water energy have good endurance to bear and keep patience.

Someone I know suffered from piles because of being seated for practice for many years and, not long after having surgery, discharge started to secrete. His doctors said that it would be better soon but he contacted me to get some advice, having some kind of bad vibes. I told him to take bamboo salt and gave some natural folk remedies and he was a little bit worried to take bamboo salt because of its salty taste.

The widespread recognition on salt is as follows. People involved in modern medicine or the general public have a prejudice that salt is mainly responsible for illnesses in kidney and liver and almost all of diseases of the time like diabetes as well as cardiovascular ones. Even in the field of modern medicine, however, they present research papers claiming that proper intake of salt is healthier. It is no need to limit intake of salt excessively except for those who are with severe high blood pressure.

The bamboo salt, in particular, is made at 1300 – 1500°C as pottery is baked so their unhealthy toxicity is already baked out. So it is seemingly salt but it can be called rather lump of heat itself. It was recently reported that Korean kimchi[16] was of anticancer effect and, among various types of kimchi, it was told that kimchi made with bamboo salt was the most effective. People make a fuss about it as if it was a groundbreaking discovery but, actually, it is common sense for those who understand natural remedies or principles or oriental medicine. Have you heard of a cancer in heart? Cancers like coldness so people with cold body should be careful not to get cancer.

To analyze the reason why so many people get cancer these days based on my clinical experience and natural principles, it is because more and more people eat sweeter and cooler food. To eat sweet and cool things causes lack of water in our bodies.

---

16) Kimchi is a traditional fermented Korean side dish made of vegetables such as napa cabbage, radish, scallion, or cucumber and with a variety of seasonings include salt, pepper, salted fish, and garlic.

When bodies lack water, dehydration occurs. It means, in other words, desertification of body. The desertification makes people dry and emotionally drained. How can people who are emotionally drained show their mercy to others? If they become so drier that they cannot shed tears, their bodies also become as stiff as their minds. People with the stiff body easily have fracture or bones with holes in them, which can cause osteoporosis or degenerative arthritis.

In terms of principles of Five Elements, lack of the water energy can cause pus or infection easily and if it it's the case, the water energy can be supplemented by eating foods with natural salty taste such as beans or bamboo salt.

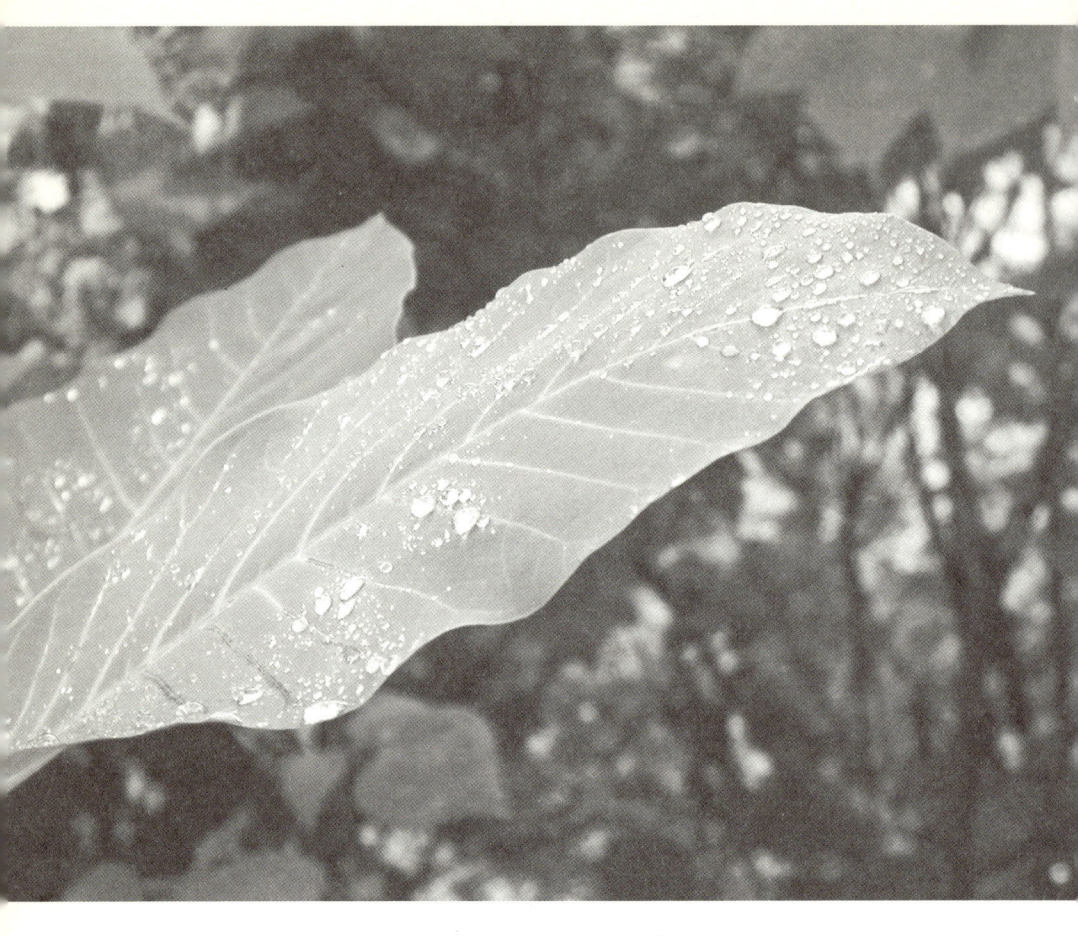

We can understand that
all energies forming us are ultimately
from the universe and the nature.

When Stomach Meets Meat

The grain not only plays a very significant role in stabilizing constitution but helps to soften energy and develop humans' spirituality.

As I have emphasized several times, what forms constitution is energy and the most important thing in the process of making constitution is environment. Above all, the most important things in the environment are water and air.

The quickest way to destroy humans' vital activities is to suffocate and to stop providing water. These two, therefore, can be called absolute condition to maintain our lives. The reason why modern people cannot make a complete use of their inborn energy is that breathing to generate energy and heaven and earth, the source of foods, are ailing. It is also a reason for people's hardheartedness and drained minds.

Unfortunately, however, water, air and environment are energies with absolute need to strengthen our vitality while we can seldom make them subject to our will. From a view of personal dimension, therefore, we should find out what can be subject to our will and care about them at least. Among elements forming energy, what we can easily change in relative sense includes dieting, practice, sleep, surrounding environment ^{living space, human relations, etc.}, sans souci and so on. Let's look into how to select and eat foods through natural ways fit for one's constitution.

Dieting is important because foods make original power for our bodies. There is a Korean saying that we live on the power from rice. This means we cannot exert energies when the harmony between Yin and Yang and dieting in our bodies is broken. Biologically, the first thing we eat after weaning is grain and the last thing at our death bed is also grain. Koreans traditionally have put soaked rice and coins in the mouth of a person who died. This symbolically indicates that it is the most important thing in a human's life to fill one's energy with grain by connecting birth and death. The grain not only plays a very significant role in stabilizing constitution but helps to soften energy and develop humans' spirituality.

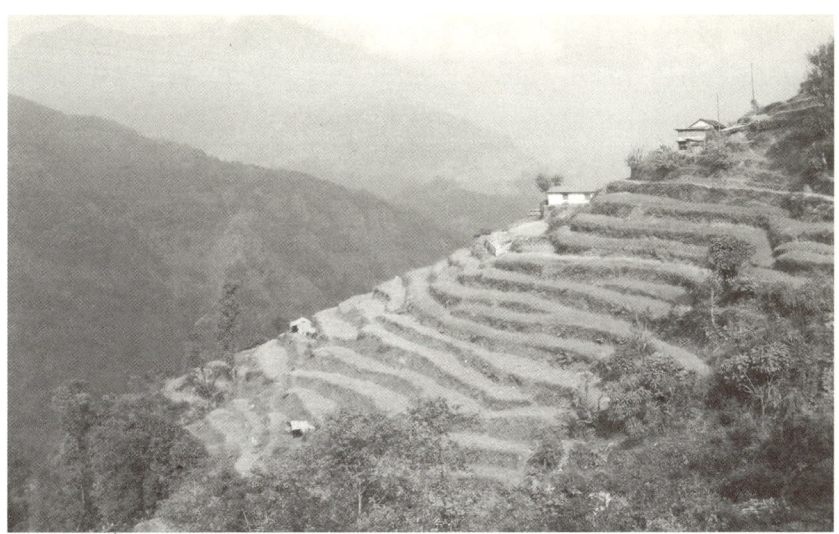
Terraced farm where the nature is alive yet in Nepal

For right dieting, you should eat natural foods mainly with grains according to your constitution. The food culture these days, however, makes light of grain and goes extremely toward meats or fruits and vegetables. Straightforwardly, taking too many fruits and vegetables makes the body cold. The body made cold means a stiffened body, which makes metabolic capability and the amount of exercise go down and the lacking amount of exercise weakens activities of cells. The weakened activities of cells are more likely to cause infections and deteriorated infections can develop into tumors or cancers. People think that fruits and vegetables cannot be eaten too much because they are rich in vitamins and fibers and they clean the blood. So fruits and vegetables are socially being recommended but taking too much of them can cause your body to be cold. Therefore, fruits and vegetables should be taken with grains.

Even with the same food, the process of digestion, absorption, storage and excretion varies according to system of one's five viscera and the six entrails. In terms of the bodily system, it takes more than double the time to digest meats than grains, which indicates that meats stay in the body that much longer. This means it takes several times of energy to digest meats than grains and it aggravates fatigue in the five viscera and the six entrails that much.

The stomach is inclined to consider all foods as enemy. Imagine yourself as the stomach. You're home alone and someone rings the bell. Can you just open the door without identifying if you think the person is not one of your family members? You will take a look on what is going on wondering who the person is. If a woman is home alone and a mail comes, she wouldn't open the door wide but take the mail through a crack with the door being latched. It is natural to have wariness to strangers. When mother says 'I'm home' outside the door, however, we quickly open the door for her in joy. Wouldn't we look through what she bought and search for something to eat? The stomach is the same. It works with the same system.

As the first thing of a newborn baby is to meet its mother, the very next thing to stomach after mother's milk is grain. The grain is the food of the least resistance to our body. The body is supposed to look for what is the most comfortable and familiar. For example, it would be grain, kimchi, cubed radish kimchi, soybean paste and red pepper paste to the body structure of our Koreans. So we come to want those things in couple of days while staying in foreign country no matter how full we are.

To get back to situation of the stomach, it is on an alert that 'Oh, this is strange' when something unfamiliar comes in. And then it secretes gastric juice to beat off the foreign substance by all means. In this circumstance, the gastric juice can be considered a kind of poison. The poison usually reminds us of that in solenoglyph or something like potassium cyanide but this poison from stomach is to ripen foods. When we cannot make gastric juice for ourselves, therefore, we take stomach medicine. This is substitute for natural gastric juice, which is the same principle that kids go and tell their mother or older brothers when they cannot beat off their enemies.

However, the thing that stomach is alert for the most is the meats. The stomach needs a tremendous amount of gastric juice and bile to digest the meats. While Westerners have short intestine appropriate for intake of meats compared to their body frame, we Asians have about one-meter-longer intestine than that of Westerners on average because we have lived mostly on grains for a long time. For bodies mainly living on grains, it takes much longer to digest meats so it can be more burdensome. Eating meats can boost up momentary power like animals but it also can deaden other precious values like patience, endurance, persistence and spirituality. When people are properly filled with energy from grains, they can have root energy and concentration and the concentration is a must for meditation. It is obvious how children will grow up only eating steak every day. So meats should be taken only with the least amount of grains, vegetables and fruits.

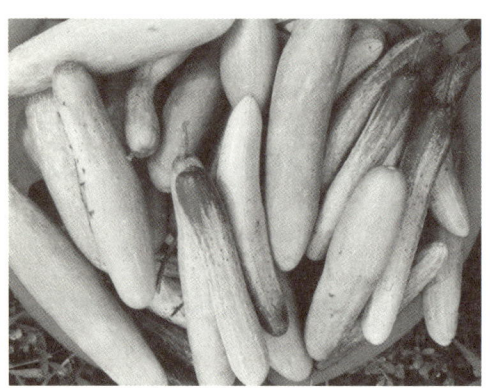

Our spirits are heavily affected by what we eat. Recall that most of carnivores get cold-bloodedly cruel in front of their prey. Animals raised in a pen forcibly are cruelly killed regardless of their will. In the process of slaughter, therefore, those animals are killed with regrets. How an animal could ever leave a will or pray that 'I am offering my body for the sake of all people's health' while being killed? Their regrets do not just go away or disappear. They are invisible but they are surely out there. That can be invisible toxicity of meats. The more we enjoy flesh of other creatures, the more alike our consciousness gets. It will make us devoted to our instinct for survival but hard to have gentle mind to others. We can take meats a little when we are physically exhausted or we need to strengthen our energy. Depending on cases, meats can be more of help to our bodies than medicines. What I want to point out here is the today's food culture which goes wrong toward excessive intake of meats and people's gluttony in it. We can generate power more than we eat only when we return to natural appetite and we are free from the gluttony.

From a yogic perspective, eating foods is not only about meeting appetite but it is a concept of energy. It is to absorb energy – Prana[17] which is wide-spread in universe – as the form of food. To seek the right well-being, what we eat matters but, more importantly, how we eat counts. The principle of the conservation of energy is also applied in eating. We should understand how to exert maximum energy out of what we eat.

---

17) It means 'breath, life and energy,' 'air and wind' in a worldly way and 'cosmic vitality' as a sacred meaning.

In that sense, natural foods are ones to generate energy the most effectively with relatively small quantity. One of advantages of eating natural foods is to make body light. In addition, it is also under control considering one's constitution and the present energy. They generate more energy with less quantity and the body comes to have less work in digestion and excretion, which makes body only lighter. This is also the reason why old disciplinants used to live mainly on grains. It is because grains have original vitality to move up the root energy.

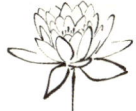

Mechanism of Cold and Cough

The cough is lungs' struggle to spit out the cold energy with all your force and measures to save yourself for your lungs.

Why do we cough or catch cold more in fall or in-between seasons than in the cold winter? It is because our bodies have the immune system against cold air in winter which has run through fall but we are not ready for air of fall which is neither cold nor hot. Strong government organizations in a town signify systems which are properly built and organized. Without such systems, we cannot but lose our precious life and property at the scene of flood or fire.

The nose hair and mucus warms air which is colder than body temperature and filters foreign waste in the air. When we stay out for enjoying night breeze in fall for a long time, however, the cool energy gradually comes into through our nostrils. The coolness is a state of hot and cold energies subtly mixed. Among those energies mixed, a piece of cold energy which is not warmed enough goes directly into lungs by passing through nose hair as if it were saying 'Catch me if you can,' wouldn't lungs be anything but startled? The lungs would be knocked down at once without any defense plan because the cold air to which they are not accustomed is suddenly coming in.

As we know, we catch a cold not because of getting cold air for a while but mainly because of suddenly breathing in cold air. At that moment, lungs proclaim alert system and strive to generate heat autonomously, which makes cough. The cough is lungs' struggle to spit out the cold energy with all your force and measures to save yourself for your lungs.

Everybody catches a cold several times and coughs but I think not many of them have thought about why they cough. It is the same as you don't have a critical mind on the reason for practice while you perform asana[18] such as histapadasana or matsyasana every day. To quickly stop coughing, the body should be warmed first. The easiest way is to wear a mask. The mask filters cold air

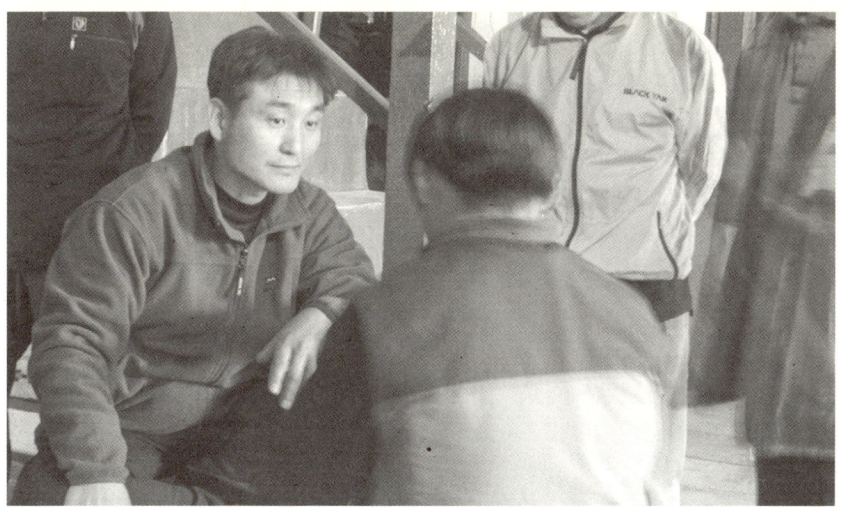

The author consulting a native about his health on the pilgrimage to Annapurna in the Himalayas

in place of the weakened nose.

Moreover, people misunderstand false heat generated by a cold as true heat and they drink cold water and have cold dishes. And they complain that they cannot get over the cold. Over a week of cold, we come to have some phlegm in throat. If the cold hasn't gone even after another week, infection comes in. The phlegm is the stage before this infection. This phlegm originally is body

---

18) It means 'movement, pose and posture' and it is also methods of actual yoga practice. According to Patanjali's Yoga Sutra, it is the third step in eight stages of yoga.

fluid but, with a cold, it is excreted with lumps of cells dead from fighting against cold virus. The dead cells should be eliminated for the body to immediately send in new recruits. When the new recruits cannot easily win the battle, people go to see a doctor for medicine at the end.

The medicine injected through, compared to modern war, functions as a missile. The missile flies off to viruses at the target spot and completely eradicates them. As we saw in Gulf War, however, missiles do not destroy targets only but burn its surroundings to the ground so historic heritages are demolished and civilians are massacred. The injected medicine works the same. It kills functioning cells around infected ones and leaves many injuries great and small and aftereffects. So when people recover in a month after all of the sufferings by inevitably going to a hospital and getting injection and medicine, they already get dead tired, which is the state of being totally worn out. It is of no use to try to take people who are totally worn out to some place nice. The only solution is to eat and rest well.

However, people do not fully understand the concept of eating well. It is not about eating bone soup or beef-rib soup. When having those dishes, we still need grains in body. While being totally worn out, we need to console cells gently with grains and wash off injuries. If possible, colds had better be treated at the very beginning and approached with natural therapies rather than medicines, which leaves fewer injuries and aftereffects on our bodies.

Modern people increasingly misuse and abuse medicines and antibiotics and they more often undergo an operation than ever before so the natural flow of energy inside the body is often changed as environment is polluted. Particularly, the abuse of antibiotic of modern people is nothing new. This is actually a very dangerous tendency. People are used to taking medicines and getting injections even for a weak cold. The more we depend upon medicines, however, the more of them we need with a tolerance, which eventually leads to immunity to drop.

Having operations and taking medicines change vitality in energies and meridians, the Yin and Yang energies in our body. Organ resection and operations which damage brains and imdok-mac (conception vessel and governor vessel), GV20 (Governor Vessel-20) and the perineum – the interface of centers at the top and the bottom – can be considered the worst in terms of bodies. The governor vessel goes down the spine from head to coccyx and the conception vessel is with the same route on the front side of the body. According to oriental medicine, our bodies cannot make good use of energies when the conception and governor vessels are damaged by lumbar operations, celioscope, cesarean or surgeries on uterus, perineal region or chest. In those cases, energy meridians, flow of Yin and Yang, do not work properly and have obstacles so energies cannot last long, which naturally lowers the power of execution in anything. Some people should receive operations inevitably. However, those who have surgeries on their center of the body would feel that they cannot exert themselves even though the surgery is a success. Thus, it is almost impossible to do things with those people continuously. They can be disappointed to slower progress than others from practice but they should make further efforts to keep their health.

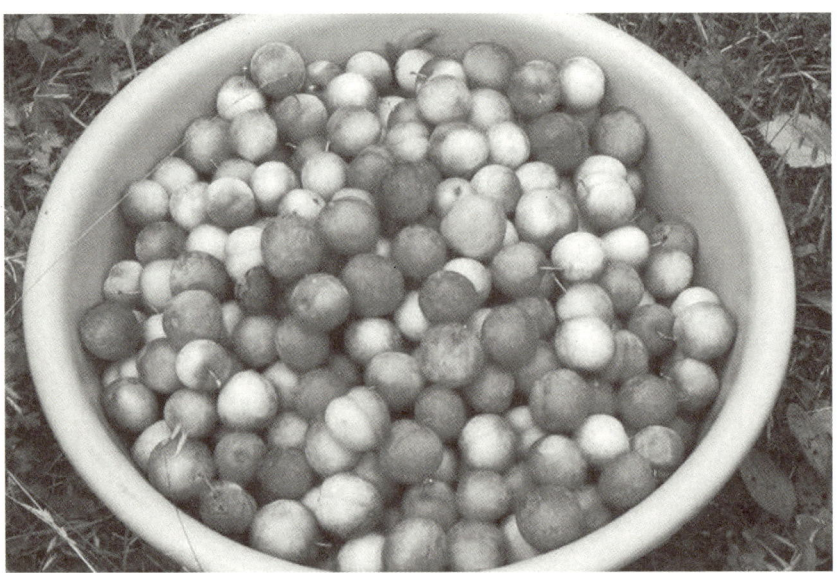

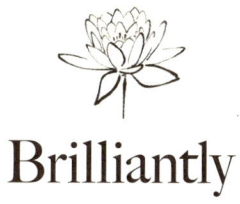

Brilliantly

When the variety of Five Elements
is well mixed as one, everything shines bright.

The five kinds in Five Elements are not only recognized as the number '5' but they are natural agency in universe classified into five big flows. For example, five grains in Five Elements from nature include wheat, sorghum and corn which have shapes stretching out and soaring into sky with the wood and fire energies. The corn, in particular, is tall and luxuriant compared to other grains as energy of mutual fire literally means the energy of diffusion. However, what about the rice representing the iron energy? As a Korean saying, it bows as it ripens. The bean with the water energy is very short in length and the yam, which has nothing to be called tall or short, grows into the ground and some of them have roots longer than one meter. In this way, Five Elements have various shapes in universe. These days, the principles of Five Elements are applied in all fields including psychotherapy, art, design, interior and architecture as well as Korean medicine, natural dieting, geomancy and naminology.

These five kinds of energies spreading in universe keep the balance in energies but sometimes are biased to one side. We Koreans use a word 'brilliantly.' When the variety of Five Elements is well mixed as one, everything shines bright. To keep this balance, Five Elements have the dynamics of the three; (i) the coexistence to one-sidedly help each other, (ii) the incompatibility to oppress and check energies unilaterally and (iii) the reversed winning to hold incompatibility.

Generally, the incompatibility is easily recognized as something bad but the incompatibility in Five Elements is not only for destruction but for maintenance of the coexistence and the reversed winning. What matters is harmony of these three – coexistence, incompatibility and reversed winning – and the structure of Five Elements cannot be properly understood if any value judgment is made like some are good while others are bad. The concept of health in terms of Oriental studies is achieved only when the five viscera and the six entrails in our bodies are well-balanced with the coexistence, incompatibility and reversed winning.

As summer is coming in, the institute where I am staying these days is full of the songs of birds. With the number of birds increasing, that of birds of prey like hawks and eagles should be increased simultaneously for the natural order in forest. To keep the ecosystem in balance, there should be hawks and eagles and then birds' singing would sound beautiful. Otherwise, all sorts of birds would warble all the time and it would be noise rather than singing.

Eating out at restaurants, we sometimes see children romping around so the restaurant gets noisy. They even run on dining tables and make us frown. In that case, the restaurant owner doesn't know what to do in the awkward situation. With this equivocal behavior, the owner may think the feelings of children's parents but overlook the fact that other customers would be lost.

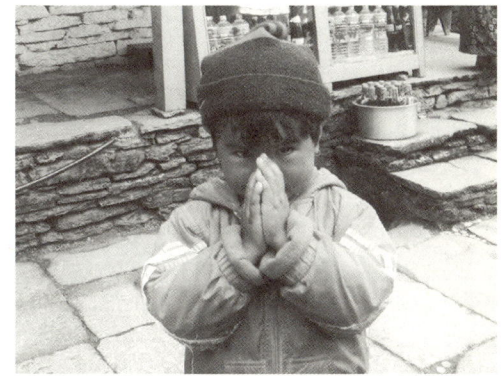

Children's being ill-mannered means there are problems in adults' educating children. If schools and parents educate children only with focusing on the coexistence, it can be the very coexistence that may actually ruin the children. To raise children as strong being, adults should make them directly experience Five Elements and be able to apply principles of the coexistence, incompatibility and reversed winning in their daily lives. Only this way, children can grow up brilliantly instead of being haughty or precocious with imitating acts of adults. The legal system also has the balance of the three powers. On trial, a lawyer should make the crime lighter or should prove innocence and a prosecutor should make the crime heavier and prove guilt. And there comes a judge who concludes through mediating the conflicting two.

The human's health is the same way. As the five viscera and the six entrails in our bodies are of organic relations with coexistence, incompatibility and reversed winning, our health is supposed to be weakened when only one of them has good or bad energy. Like this, Five Elements in our bodies and minds can be completed through harmony and balance of coexistence, incompatibility and reversed winning and we can obtain sans souci under less physical and mental stress with healthier body.

Understanding the nature harmonized in this variety is also a study topic in yoga.

Life Being Also of Principles of Screw

The study for our ancestors was to obtain life wisdom through experiencing all changes great and small in energies coming from the nature.

Fresh sprouts in spring shoot up with spiral form, not with one of straight line. All the changing energies head with spiral form in which straight lines and curves move together. Look at a bullet. It seems to move in a straight line but it actually flies in an arc. Even that swift bullet is of a structure that cannot make it go forward in a straight line. In all energies' sweeping in and out, a structure of a straight line does not exist. Isn't it the reason why a screw once hammered is hardly loosened because of its spiral form?

For another example, a baby being born comes out with spiral form, not in a straight line. The birth canal is only ten-centimeter-long but it is a life-and-death journey for the baby to pass through the canal. The canal is of convolution to prevent the baby from suffocation. Thus, the baby gets out the canal while twisting its body side to side.

These phenomena are soon understood within meditation. The spiral structure where straight lines and curves coexist is seen in, for example, typhoons, human DNA and cakra[19], one of main concepts of yogic philosophy. Ancient disciplinants had already understood such structure through grasping natural laws and principles of energy through meditation but, in the opposite way, scientists are proving the fact with experiments these days.

The spiral structure in yoga is the energy passage called nadis. Pingala-nadi[20] and ida-nadi[21], the most important passages, swirl

---

19) It means 'wheel and circle' and the energy center located along the spine. It is said that there are major seven cakra in yoga. It is a similar concept to danjeon of the East, the lower part of the abdomen.
20) It is located on the right of sushumna and is responsible for warming up the body with being connected with the sun. It corresponds to the sympathetic nerve in modern medicine.
21) It is located on the left of sushumna and it is charge of cooling down the body with being related to cold energy of the moon. It corresponds to the parasympathetic nerve in terms of medicine.

around sushumna-nadi[22]. Actual practice of yoga largely consists of the three; asana, pranayama and meditation and asana is also of triple structure of postures done with sitting, standing and lying. In Five Elements, the circulation is performed when the three principles of coexistence, incompatibility and reversed winning are balanced. Other than these, there are many others with the triple structure like the oriental idea of Heaven-Earth-Man, the Trinity of the Father, the Son, and the Holy Spirit in Christianity and Buddha-Doctrine-Priest in Buddhism, etc. The dynamics of power is maintained with the triple structure.

The galaxy, DNA and typhoons all have the triple structure of energies coming in, naught at the center and energies going out. All phenomena in the world can be explained with this principle.

Let's compare the state of being sick to a circumstance that a screw is deeply hammered into a wall. The screw is not easily or quickly plucked out with hands and everything including the screw can be damaged. The screw should be picked out by slowly turning it. In terms of principles, therefore, the more se-

---

22) It is a central passage getting up with spine to the crown of the head and leads immortality. Pingala-nadi and ida-nadi are twisting around this.

rious a disease is, the more it needs to get rid of a root cause instead of covering up visible phenomena for a while simply with some medicines. It is especially required for lingering or serious diseases. By starting to solve big and visible problems first, our energies are gradually restored in the process of Five Elements turning round and round while the body's autogenous power gradually revives.

The process of getting healthy through practice is the same. What feels good at the beginning can bring about unexpected symptoms or sore spots according to one's condition over time with various additional effects. In other words, as blocked spots where circulation has not been active are penetrated, the body goes through tumultuous changes and it stores up energies to get on the next stage. The additional effects occur during this process.

In general, the additional effects are developed during the period of adjustment for a disease to be cured. If these additional effects are not properly accepted, one cannot enter the next stage of health. The feeling of physical improvement is always with energies and the feeling of discomfort is from energies' temporal rest for adjustment in the body. These processes indicate that our bodies go along the flow as we speak out sometime and step back some other times. So, even when the additional effects are

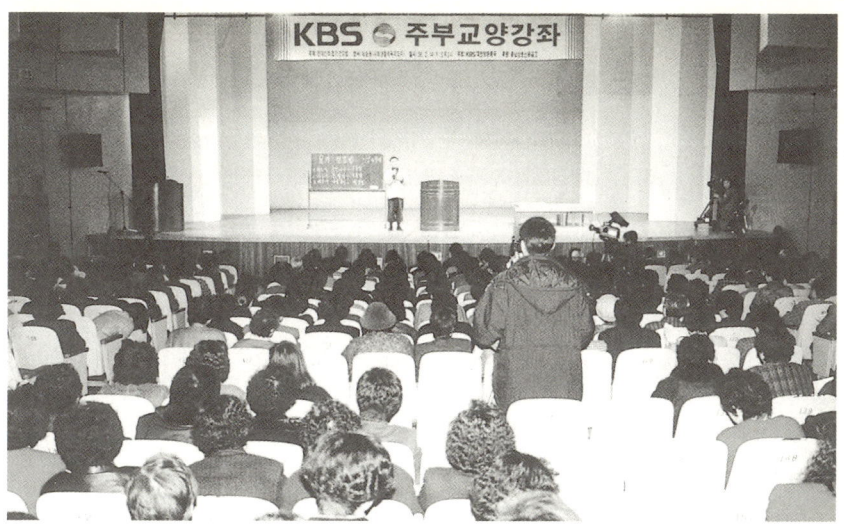

The author on the lecture in KBS(Korea Broadcasting System)

gone and you feel better a little, you never let the guard down but get fully prepared for the next stage not to give up against all odds. The process of physical improvement is to identify gradual progress through the repetition of energies gathered and relaxed while they turn round and round in the five viscera and the six entrails.

An old saying goes that ten years is an epoch. This refers to the fact that Five Elements of nature are changing on a ten-year cycle. Among the Five Elements of *mok* (wood), *hwa* (fire), *to* (earth), *keum* (iron) and *su* (water), there is a year when one of them exceeds and lacks so those elements come and go in turn.

If this year is with excessive water energy, the next year will be with weak wood energy and the year after next is with strong fire energy. In this way, Five Elements come and go twice with being strong and weak for a decade. Thus I have considered a decade as the cycle for studying as it has been said that at least ten years is required to specialize in something.

The study for our ancestors was to obtain life wisdom through experiencing all changes great and small in energies coming from the nature. If we haven't studied enough yet and we can't understand the power of nature on ourselves, we can't wisely deal with different circumstances in life. People feel so much energetic in one year and waste the energy being overwhelmed by it. They feel so depressed in another year and they get way too pessimistic about the world drinking and complaining that nothing is working out. So they are called foolish, instead of being wise. In a year with excessive energy, it should be reserved and in another year with weak energy, you can handle the circumstances based on principles by studying what you need.

The life is the same. When we are successful, we save money for a rainy day and oblige others who are going through difficult times. And we come to receive help from them when we are placed in a difficult situation later. That's the way our life goes, right? The principles in all lives are like that of a screw.

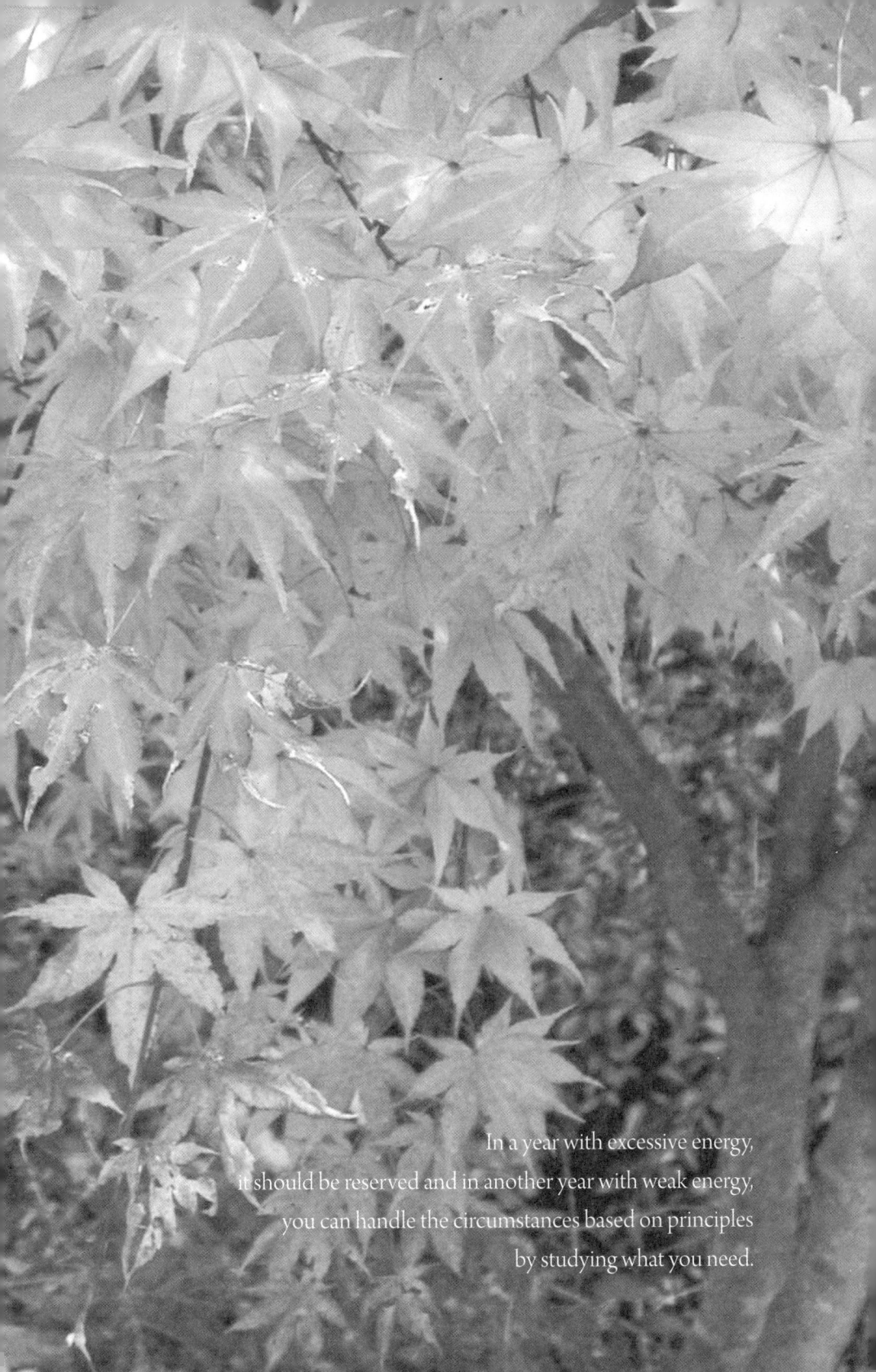

In a year with excessive energy,
it should be reserved and in another year with weak energy,
you can handle the circumstances based on principles
by studying what you need.

Contemplation on Vitality

We can display our vitality bursting from the inside
only with our firsthand behavior and practice.

Being so-called diesel has been a social issue these days. Men keep lifting weight to make six-pack and women constantly lose their weight and some immature women have breast enlargement operations for people's saying bigger breasts are attractive to men.

As you are well aware, however, being diesel doesn't mean people who are physically healthy but who have model-like figure. Paying attention to one's own body is a good thing but it is problematic that the attention is with a structure of being obsessed with absurd images made by media and capital. The bodies built up this way is not harmonized with one's mind but degenerated into a means to show off and to satisfy their desire for ostentation. Their goal is not to make the body healthier but they just overdo themselves to have the body fit into a socially acknowledged standard for physical beauty. Do you know that some bodybuilding champions use muscle enhancing supplements and many other drugs who brag to others about their six-pack and the muscular big-built and some women champions have operations at the risk of their life? These phenomena indicate that our society does not have philosophy or true experience on the body.

Look at the students of nowadays. They simply do not have time to play around or exercise being busy studying whether they are in elementary, middle or high school. During the children's period of growth, they need activities appropriate for physical growth to have well balanced mind and body when they grow up. They surely need exercise as their bodies get bigger but they just study sitting at their desk so the healthy energy for life activities cannot come out and the body is off-balance, which sets their nerves on edge. What will they be like when they become adults? The bodies left without any exercise until their middle or high school days cannot restore the balance even with all measures after being fully grown and they come to be obsessed only with its appearance.

In one's 20s, consciousness should be raised instead of physical growth. Being immature is a state of a full-grown body without the mind getting mature. Look at how a child grows into an adult. For the first one year after birth, they remarkably grow physically. Over the adolescence, the rate of physical growth gradually decreases and it generally stops around the age of twenty. That is how a body works. The physical growth is of course the most dramatic as a fetus because that process is to make something out of nothing only with a seed of life. Babies born as 3kg on average require tremendous energy to make its body at least several times bigger for a year. That is why they make fanatical efforts to suck their mother's breast. Thus, the first-birthday party is to celebrate their efforts and praiseworthy behaviors for growth and expansion in the meantime.

Children's energies mostly have energy of mutual fire [Simpo and Samcho23)] in general Simpo and Samcho are concepts similar to the

---

23) According to oriental medicine, there are Simpo and Samcho which are invisible organs connecting the five viscera and the six entrails. Simpo functions as prime minister or liege assisting heart, the sovereign of five viscera and Samcho circulates energies by handling all of functions such as digestion, absorption, excretion and breathing. These two are called the energy of mutual fire based on Five Elements.

autonomic nerve in occidental medicine. Therefore, when the energies of Simpo and Samcho come out, it means the nerve system is instable, energies in five viscera and six entrails are disturbed and the body loses its balance. When the balance in head or body is broken, anyone comes to have the energies of Simpo and Samcho. For children, they instinctively have data input for growth and they have Simpo and Samcho because their energies are intensively used for basic life activities like eating and excreting.

However, after their physical growth is completed in some degree and Five Elements in their body are fairly under way naturally, their energies of Simpo and Samcho are gradually stabilized. What matters is when energies of Simpo and Samcho are still made and these energies mainly used for urgent life activities. Simpo and Samcho in children are considered necessary for physical growth but those energies in adults are not regarded as a normal state. People who have gone through operations or medication surely have these energies because of disturbance in nerve system. Otherwise, the phenomenon can be explained that it comes from imbalance of body and mind. For

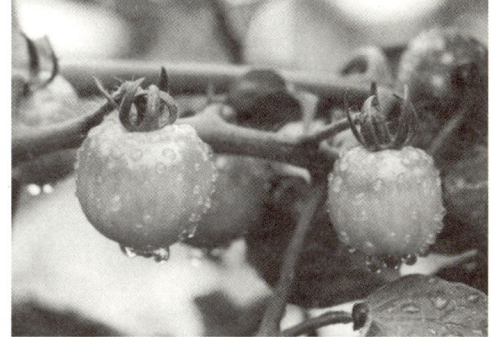

example, people subject to this circumstance may have studied hard but have little experience on body or they seldom work with their head but do a lot of physical activities only.

For businesses, it would be better to employ people with strong ability to maintain their livelihood who have grown up and studied in underprivileged surroundings over other people with excellent academic record and backgrounds who are poor at practice as a Korean saying goes 'It is a hawk that catches a pheasant.' It means, unfortunately, our society is entirely going with such a structure. We cannot do as much as we know and we don't know what to do. Isn't it that we live only theoretically without practice?

On the other hand, too much physical training without studying or reading is also a problem. It is particularly troublesome when those people launch forward to be a yoga teacher. In this case, there is nothing we can do. In terms of spirit and material and the perspective of Yin and Yang, that is called the disorder.

We have vitality only when the mind and body are balanced. Those who are biased toward either theories or physical training cannot have creativity. For example, we cannot paint or play instruments well when we have knowledge only on art and music.

We can display our vitality bursting from the inside only with our firsthand behavior and practice. Beyond thinking, we should stretch our ideas and arts through the sensitive sense on our fingertips and constant footwork.

Thus, I think today's education should be focused more on field practice. What is more important than solving math problems and memorizing English words is watching how a flower blooms and how rice we eat is grown and thinking why the air and the water is important themselves. Being free from a room to read a plant book and to memorize names of plants, they should set off exploration for plants everywhere, getting around through the mountains.

We don't get excited only to see flowers in a book. We feel our heart beating upon encounter with things alive in person and then we can start communicating with them through our entire senses mobilized. People who see the flower in person cannot forget the inspiration and come to write poetry, draw a picture or compose music on the flower. We also should have affection that way. We should love others wholeheartedly instead of calculating in our head. Our lives should go that way. We should constantly communicate with other existence through practical and specific actions in addition to intellectual understanding as a concept. In that way, we should meet up other creatures alive.

Practice to be Exact and Practical

*Practice brings you a number of failure and success.
The failure and success makes Yin and Yang
so if you observe what the circulation of your failure
and success means in everyday practice, the day will come
when our small and weak seed becomes the universe.*

I once talked with a Buddhist priest who had been a chief priest at a temple. He said that there was another priest who made others uncomfortable even with his asceticism over for ten years. He said maybe the priest was too much devoted to practicing and it rather caused some kind of obsession. Yes. What matters in practicing is not how long you've been practicing. Only with obsessions and thoughts developed just sitting even for a decade of practicing asceticism, we can get only tense and sensitive with excessive Yang energy[24] in our bodies.

Having many thoughts, for example, is a phenomenon developed by a disease in spleen and stomach, the earthen organs and people come to have unrealistic thinking with illnesses in the earthen organs. Meditation is practical and concrete so it shouldn't be that way. Some people utter meaningless words while their minds go wrong during meditation. For proper practice of meditation in particular, people should first understand the principle of bodies and have wisdom to rule their bodies according to the root energy of their own and the practice should be performed practically.

What does the practical practice mean? The word 'practical' should not be misunderstood as astute behaviors. Is it practical if one thinks that he will practice two hours tomorrow after skipping today's practice? It would make sense only when he practices whole day after skipping a week. It is not a practical relationship even between friends that I treat friends today so I'll be treated tomorrow. In swinging one's arm during the practice, some people's faces are twitching. That is because their heart is stimulated when swinging arms and the stimulus is conveyed to facial muscles which are related to the heart. Some would say they have nothing on their faces even after thirty times of swing.

---

24) A state of excitement

Then I tell them to swing thousand times and see if their faces wouldn't twitch even at that moment. Nothing can be concluded before reaching the extremity. If you don't feel get better even with practice, you haven't practiced hard enough to get to the threshold for enhancing your level of health. Still, you shouldn't get the yoga disease with too much obsession on yoga itself.

In practicing, some people have pain on elbows or on the entire body depending on one's health. This means that our bodies are in a chaotic state. The region where we feel pain is subject to coldness. Because of the coldness, we get stiff as a dead body is rigid and stiff because it doesn't have warmth. If we cannot overcome the pain, numbness comes in and then paralysis. When the paralysis is on heart, it is heart attack and it becomes stroke and cerebral hemorrhage on brain. We should cure the pain lest it develops into paralysis. Untangling our bodies through practice is to make the body flexible and soft so that we can lengthen our breath. On the contrary, the breathing shortens when our bodies get stiff.

So does the consciousness. For changes in consciousness, physical exercise and shock to the consciousness are required. I don't mean it is physical shock that is necessary for awakening of consciousness. Even with the physical shock, people who have clear consciousness can understand why they are hit at the moment of hitting. It is totally different from a response upon hitting like "Why are you hitting?" Wouldn't the Great Master Seosan have been enlightened at a moment when a totally different dimension of consciousness came to him?

Likewise, the responses during the practice such as twisted muscles and tendons and movements in the nerve system should not be recognized as physical shock. When we are on the flow of those responses, energies are exchanged and changed, which leads to even cells to be awakened. To perform asana only with physical force is fundamentally different from doing it along with breathing. With breathing, it leads our bodies. It may sound unreasonable but that kind of experience is indescribable. So there is no other way but to experience personally. This is the practicality I'm saying.

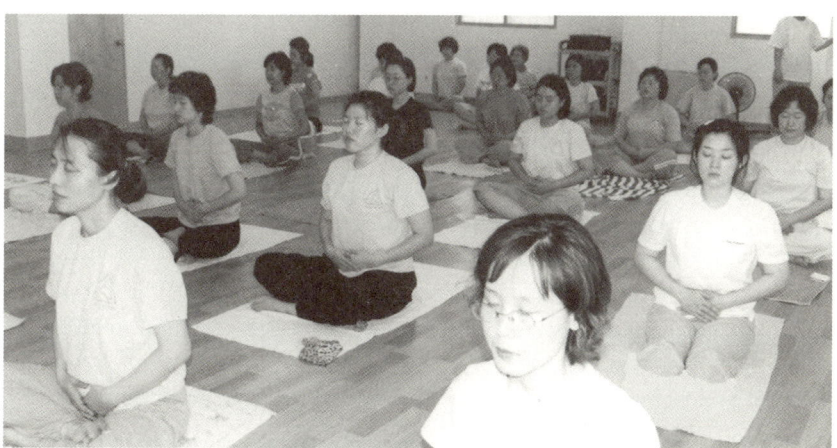

As mentioned several times before, principles handed down without experiments on bodies cannot be digested as one's own and an ability to confront stress and physical strength cannot but decrease. When we are tired and stressful, the breathing is dragged by movements and so is consciousness by the body. A lump of knowledge, not wisdom, drags us down. We should make the consciousness lead breathing and the breathing lead the body.

Good postures are not determined by your flexibility. We do not practice to be a frog. If you ever wanted to be a frog, eat up a number of snakes during this life. Then wouldn't you be born as a frog to be eaten by a snake in the life next with karma[25] of preying on so many snakes?

Let's assume that you complete Pascimottanasana. Then you don't have to practice this asana ever again? The completion this time guarantees that you will be able to perform the movement anytime? As days and nights occur, the body also stiffens if you do not practice the movement. But it is also a wrong thinking

---

25) It generally means actions and conscious actions in a deeper sense. It is related to individual's mental force in intention, thinking and actions and it is sometimes regarded as destiny determined by quality of former and present lives.

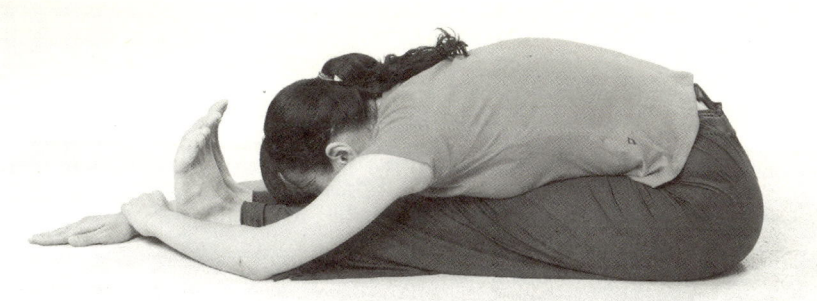
Pascimottanasana

that you don't have to practice because someday your body will stiffen anyway. Not doing anything more exhausts you. Your body gradually improves while it stiffens and relaxes repeatedly.

Practice brings you a number of failure and success. The failure and success makes Yin and Yang so if you observe what the circulation of your failure and success means in everyday practice, the day will come when our small and weak seed becomes the universe.

To live with mentally boosted values makes us physically less tired and to work with the flow of consciousness gives us wisdom not to choose a tiring way in our lives. The deeper our movements and breathing becomes, the more difficult movements we can perform and further, we can control difficult problems in life with consciousness. Through these procedures, we come to have true changes in body and mind.

In doing yoga, you should constantly ask yourself whether you are intensely agonizing to be independent from existing old notions and authority. As we cannot avoid personal hardship in our lives, we shouldn't extremely drive problems into a corner impatiently but have an attitude of the consciousness adjusted by deep and slow breathing to follow the flow and the law of nature.

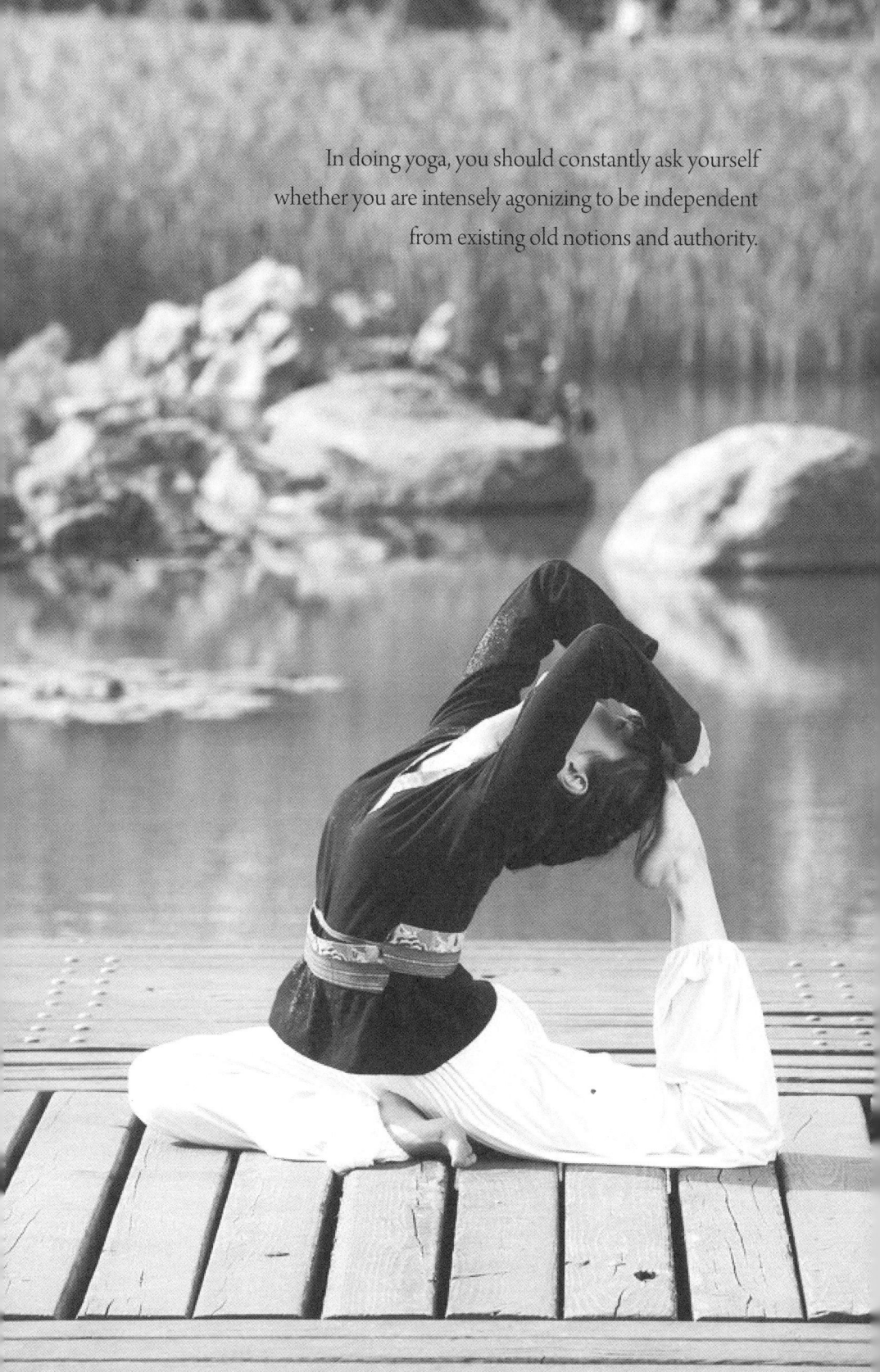

In doing yoga, you should constantly ask yourself whether you are intensely agonizing to be independent from existing old notions and authority.

Yoga, Trapped in Alternative Medicine

When we were kids and had stomachache,
wouldn't it be gone soon with grandmother's hands stroking our belly saying
'My hands are healing hands?'

Until recently, it has seemed that there is an equation of 'Yoga = Diet' but these days yoga appears to be included in concepts like natural healing and alternative medicine which are booming nowadays. Personally, I am a little unhappy with this trend.

The concepts of natural healing and alternative medicine are all from American way of thinking. Occidental medicine draws what is not understood even with cutting edge medical techniques into its field with those concepts and just recognizes them as secondary means to fill in limitations of the occidental medicine.

What is interesting is that those alternative remedies they are now using originally were our main natural remedies. Recall a piece of your childhood memory. When we were kids and had stomachache, wouldn't it be gone soon with grandmother's hands stroking our belly saying 'My hands are healing hands?' Though we think it as an uncivilized and countrified thing but it is a direct example of the natural healing. This can also be explained with the principle of yoga. The important energy center in our bodies is called cakra and we have manipura cakra in the abdomen. This flame of this manipura cakra burns and digests what we eat so we are likely to have indigestion and stomachache if we have a cold stomach. We don't have stomachache and digest foods well with the hands stroking the belly.

The reason why our way of thinking comes to have western frame mainly is the Christianity. It was severely persecuted in its early days as it collided with home-brew and shamanist elements rooted in every single Korean. Going through Japanese occupation[26] and Korean War[27], however, it could significantly expand

---

26) Annexed dependency of the Empire of Japan(1910-1945)
27) The Korean War (25 June 1950 – 27 July 1953) was a war between the Republic of Korea (South Korea), supported by the United Nations, and the Democratic People's Republic of Korea (North Korea), at one time supported by the People's Republic of China and the Soviet Union.

in political and economic chaos. For its background, influence from American Christianity was dominant which was in line with logic of market. Thus, Korean intellectuals cannot easily get out of its influence. For example, Seoul National University does not have a department of oriental medicine. If we do not make a go of acupuncture in oriental medicine or natural remedies ourselves, we would have to go to America or the West for studies of the East.

Yoga is a general and integrated philosophy encompassing partial and peripheral things. It doesn't deserve to be regarded as a secondary thing put in something else like alternative medicine or healing. Yoga is actually a great thing so it is such a pity that some yoga people mention yoga as the alternative medicine. Yoga is just yoga itself with no need of any modifiers. People return home in glory bragging that they get degree on natural healing at some university in America or India. Yoga philosophy, however, is on the premise of one's being enlightened with principles on nature and people and practicing.

In India, they have a traditional medicine called Ayurveda, which is in contrast to the modern medicine. It is a concept similar to Korean medicine of ours. Let's assume that a yoga instructor studies natural healing in America or Ayurveda in India. That kind of education can be of a little help in doing yoga but further studies and experiments are required to apply the perspective of Ayurveda to common Koreans.

It is because Ayurveda has been based on Indians' constitutional karma and a view of practice since several centuries ago. For example, it is told not to eat strong-tasting foods like garlic and red pepper powder in Ayurveda. Buddhist precepts also have o-shin-chae (five foods not to be taken) which are garlic, green onion, chives, wild chive and leeks. The reason for Ayurveda and Buddhism to forbid pungent food is that those ingredients tend to strengthen sexual function so they disturb meditation practice.

One of my close acquaintances who I've known well and who has been hard in Buddhist practice caught tuberculosis and I told him about foods to be of help. I cooked Korean native chickens in which garlic and other ingredients helpful for tuberculosis were put and gave him to have one a week. He was so shocked and felt pressured saying that he couldn't eat meats and garlic in doing practice. It was natural for him because it was to violate his religious precepts.

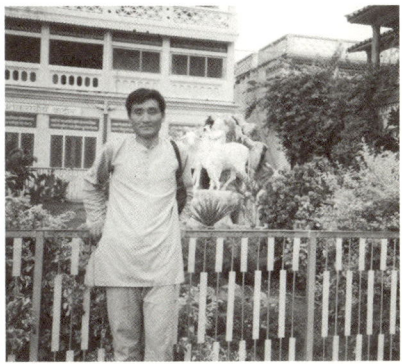
Author at a Hindu Temple in India

But, was there tuberculosis 2500 years ago when Buddhist precepts were made? Tuberculosis is one of new diseases developed during the recent two centuries and it has been tremendously spreading due to bad air in cities after the Industrial Revolution. If not taking my advice, he would have to take tuberculosis medicine for six months or even for a few years. The six-month-long medication can cause problems in stomach and disturb the nerve system as well. If a disease is acute one and gets worse rapidly, one should do whatever he or she can with any medication of East and West and dietary treatment but any therapy method too much biased to one side can be only temporary. Tuberculosis can cause partial damage in the nerve system even after being cured and it can be an obstacle in meditation with impaired concentration. The natural treatment, on the other hand, quickens recovery and has fewer side effects. Then, which would be wiser, to make energies with natural foods with one's own body or to make medicine come into the body for treatment? I am not telling you to have dichotomous thinking between taking medicines or receiving natural treatment. I mean you should make a judgment by wholly and objectively understanding and observing circumstances.

Even if we are eager to practice or meditate, it is hard with physical problems. So it is necessary to make base for practice with right diet, regulated life, moderate exercise, easy breathing and meditation.

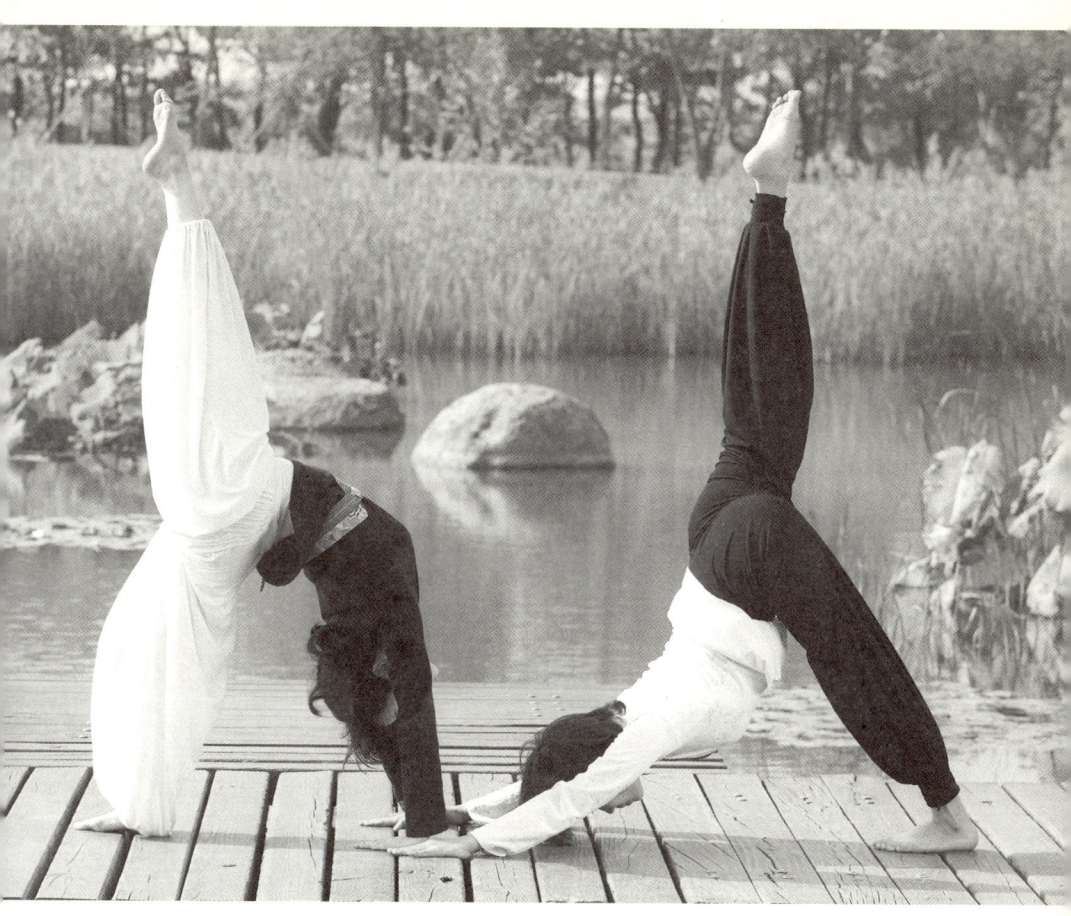

Yoga is a general and integrated philosophy encompassing partial and peripheral things.

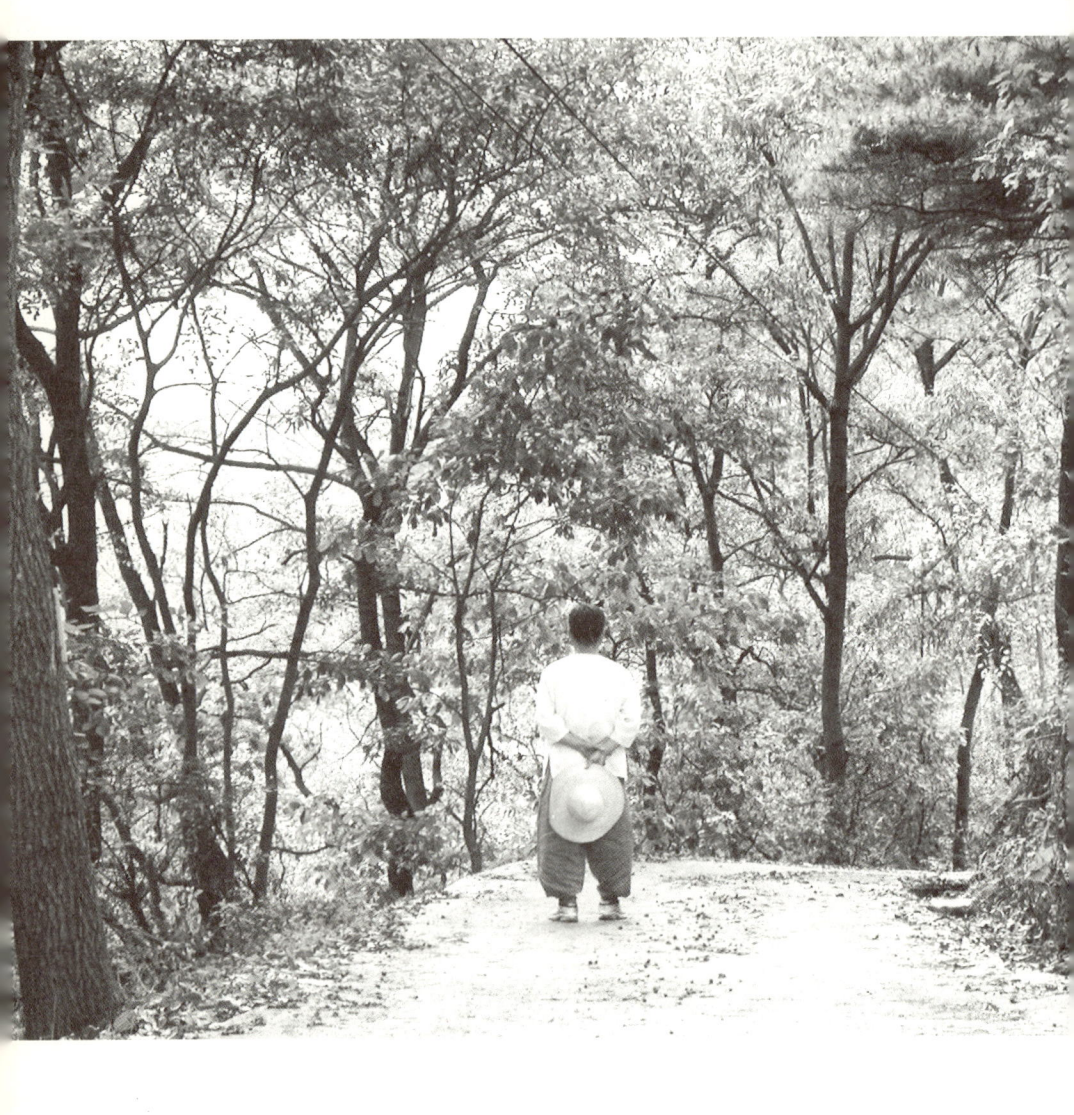

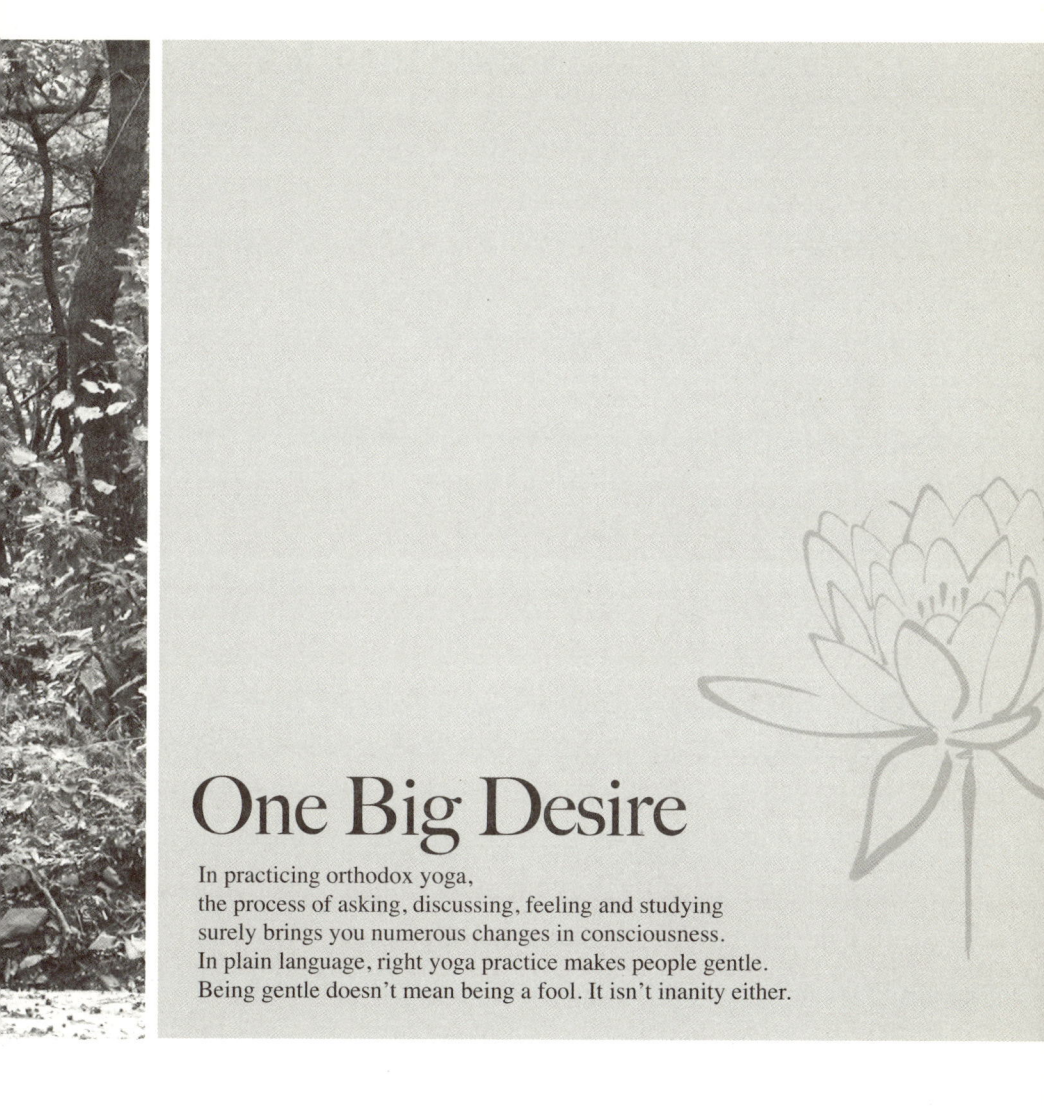

One Big Desire

In practicing orthodox yoga,
the process of asking, discussing, feeling and studying
surely brings you numerous changes in consciousness.
In plain language, right yoga practice makes people gentle.
Being gentle doesn't mean being a fool. It isn't inanity either.

Let's Have One Big Desire

Yoga is a struggle with consciousness.

Korean ideal of education is Hongik-Ingan[28]. The concept Hongik-Ingan is to extensively benefit all people. When we were young, our parents taught us to be a true human being but young parents of these days try to make their children some kind of experts. It is because they put more emphasis on being experts in a field than on being a true human being to achieve success

---

28) 'Hongik-Ingan' means extensively benefit all people.

and to get ahead in the world.

The theme of yoga is human. The best lesson for our Koreans is Hongik-Ingan. If a purpose of teaching or learning is not to benefit others, it cannot be called education. Looking into lessons of yoga, they are no different from the national spirit coming down from ancient times. They are all about respecting people and living in a harmony with neighbor. That's all.

Yoga Sutra[29] defines that yoga is to remove restlessness of mind. To study yoga is to build up life energy while you keep asking your mind getting excited and then calmed unceasingly for the entire life and self-examine yourself countless times. In practicing orthodox yoga, therefore, the process of asking, discussing, feeling and studying surely brings you numerous changes in consciousness. In plain language, right yoga practice makes people gentle. Being gentle doesn't mean being a fool. It isn't inanity either. When our body and mind are with the natural and gentle flow, we are freed from all diseases and obsessions and we can escape from anger and greed, jealousy and envy, fear and fright, arrogance and inferiority which torture our mind and emotion and which are inevitable in lives.

---

29) It is a yoga scripture with the highest authority organized by Patanjali, the father of yoga and it systematizes eight practice stages of orthodox yoga.

Yoga philosophy is that of human being. Our Koreans' ideal of education is Hongik-Ingan. As I have already mentioned several times, would any God truth, principle, law be properly treated in this world where neither are humans? This calculation is so simple. Solving too difficult and complex math problems in our lives, we seem to have forgotten simple and easy truth.

This is my principle of yoga to you. It is you can reach the level of true state of yoga that consciousness leads breathing and then breathing leads the body beyond adjusting your breath and consciousness to movements through right practice of orthodox yoga. This level of principle requires a lot of study. Therefore, the primary study for yoga teachers is practice in everyday lives.

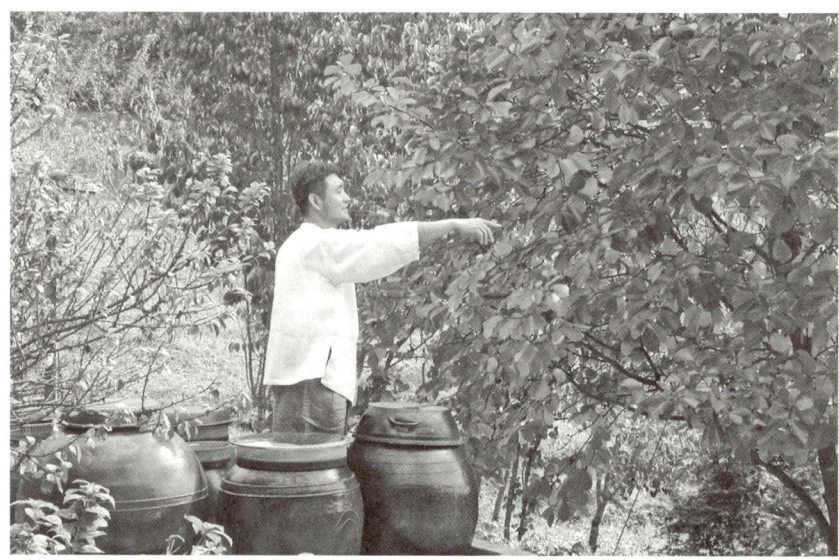

How can a yoga teacher give lessons for practice to others without his or her own practice? Practicing for cultivating one's body and mind should come first and be deepened to open up the way to true practice.

Yoga is a struggle with consciousness. The true orthodox yoga is not built overnight. When the consciousness comes at the center, the energies from yoga will always be in your life even if you do not practice for a couple of months or go to the yoga studio. Thanks to that principle of yoga, it can have been handed down for thousands of years.

If you really intend to practice yoga, particularly orthodox one, why not throw away all of secular greed but this one desire? The one to head forward to state of true yoga with deeper practice and through mastering the principle. Imagine this parascientific, supernatural and innovative body and mind that consciousness naturally leads the flow of breathing and the breading leads the body. Picture you feel the lighter body and easier breathing and mind just with capillary exercise and Savasana after getting off work as if you practiced asana for a few hours. Try learning it. Practice is not done only in studios but everything in our lives is already practice.

Believe in your body! Let go your age!

Do not care your gender! Don't be conscious of your physical and mental illnesses!

Have faith that your practice will certainly succeed!

I sincerely hope you to be independence fighters of health and wisdom.

Aum!

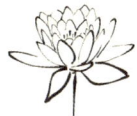

Study to be Done in One's Youth

People should work with more efforts during their youth
and should do study at every moment of everyday.
It is also important to form right habits constantly with
regular life of sleeping and getting up early.

Many people become too sensitive with unnecessary things. They quibble too much over things that are not truly theirs. That makes obsession. By contrast to that, true wisdom is not about memorization or clumsy imitation so it rises from various circumstances like spring water with no time to think or even worry.

The unwise just literally understand lessons from old sages who have conveyed truth instead of grasping them seriously.

Those who have diverse experiences can partially understand through their accumulated experience with age. That is, however, still limited understanding not being freed from personal karma based on each individual's system of consciousness so it is on a totally different dimension from borderless wisdom of those who are enlightened. Thus, it would be far more difficult for the young with less experience to even partially understand lessons from old sages. If you really intend to live a natural life and to practice, it is important to ask yourself persistently what you want to know. People who have had a true critical mind only once can understand. The entire universe is in one's body and

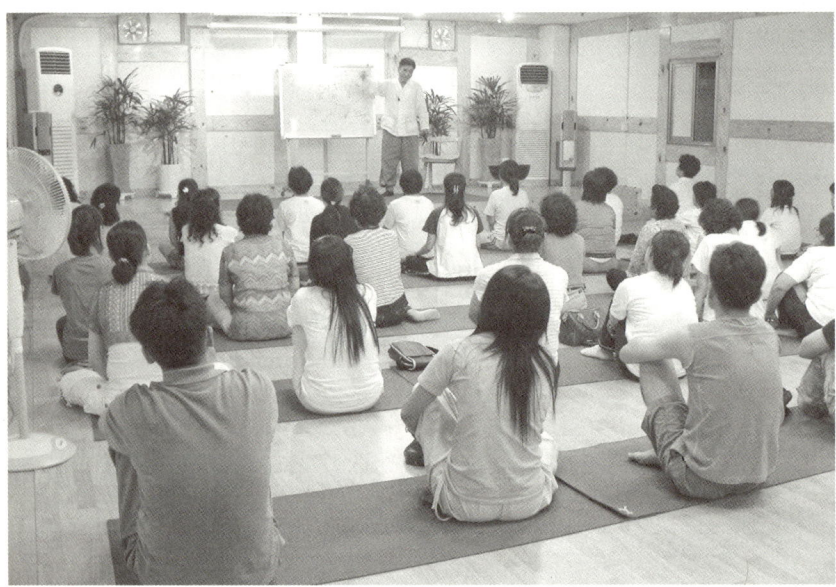

the answer is hidden in oneself as well.

Spiritual masters in history have had great courage to confront problems and wrongness in society of the day. Buddha set forth a view of equality against caste system, the deep-rooted vice in India and Jesus stood against the cruel Roman Empire barehanded.

My teaching that yoga shouldn't be chosen as one of professions would be also against the current of this modern capitalistic society. The reason why I stick to it, however, is the standard of joy in yoga is different from that of the world. People should work with more efforts during their youth and should do study at every moment of everyday. It is also important to form right habits constantly with regular life of sleeping and getting up early. This is practice within lives and it would end up as a house of cards without this basis.

Where to Go After Using Up This Body

Not understanding is because of living with the mind being closed.

I guess everyone has their own difficulties in this season changing into summer only after a slight air of spring. In one's youth, you would like to go out to mountains and plains to radiate youthfulness. No matter what kind of relationship we personally have, I cherish the all connections with you. You may feel you are somewhat young or old but you are not definitely aged at all so you may be happy and then annoyed about everything even in a single day. Wouldn't be there some meanings to bring you down here? Even one clump of grass or a bug crawling on it has its life for its own connection. Questions like where we are from before obtaining this body and where we are heading after using this up may not be only for monks up on a mountain. I have told you this several times already.

Life and principles of the world are in coexistence of relative brightness and darkness in things. We are now at an important crossroad to well preserve our spirit and to improve it further in this world of cutthroat competition. Nobody can escape from hardship if everyone thinks it's hard. What is clear, however, is that there are people who suffer from pains that you cannot even imagine. In your eyes, people who have and enjoy more material affluence would stand out.

The inner peace, however, is not visible from outside. When someone is exhausted and gives up what he or she was doing without recognizing what makes them difficult, we call it emptiness. You may not know the fact that you are going through a tremendous change in your habits before you know it. You consciousness is changing, which might be insignificant but definite. It doesn't bear complete fruits yet because it has not become sophisticated or ripe enough. Have you ever seen anyone living an idle life or thoughtlessly caring only about their bodies look after others or neighbors? Wouldn't it be right to leave this world as a human being after living a life even less worthy than that of one clump of grass?

    Have pride in yourself.
    Believe in yourself.
    Don't be excessively outraged.
    Don't envy others too much.
    And don't be eaten up with conceit.
    With close look at you like this, the hidden virtue would be greatly cultivated.

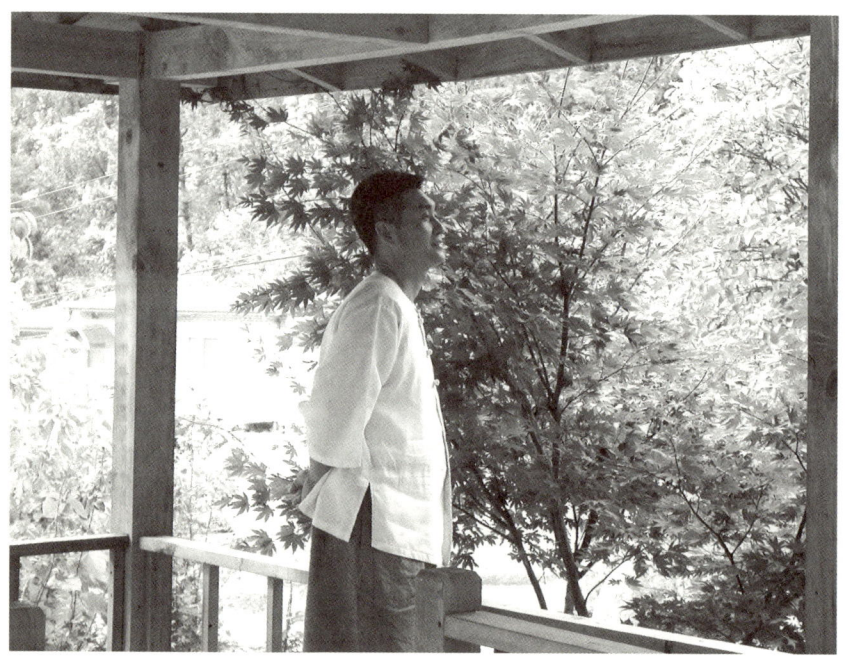

Not understanding is because of living with the mind being closed. You cannot see others with obsession about yourself. 'Others' here mean other people and the universe. Losing people around you means that a ghost^{chaos} comes in the place of them. You should fix this meaning in your mind. Losing people's heart and support, you never know what kind of hardship and difficulty you will be faced.

You are not people to teach techniques. I've never intended to foster technicians. Even now, you may constantly not understand what I'm saying but, through deep introspection, I hope you to practice meditation in every aspect of life. Ask yourself once again. Where are we heading after using up this body?

Change Yourself

To keep a good connection each other, don't try to change others but yourself.

Perhaps a life is with not so much to do. Our lives may not be a big deal in some aspects. Paradoxically, that's why we should save time. We should really cherish the time. In one-hour session to teach practice, I spend only one hour but with ten members in it, that's ten hours and with twenty, it is work to handle energies of twenty hours. I am responsible for the ten, twenty hours. You should be able to calculate this way. Would it be fair to spend the precious time irresponsibly? That's just the waste of each other's life.

Lately, we did some work on a valley in the institute and a backhoe driver tried burying the stones left after the work was over. I saw that and asked him to pile up those stones on one side and I finally rebuilt steps with them a few days ago. What I felt during this physical labor after a long time that the work was done by two in a day didn't mean I could have done it in two days for myself. It could take several days or I might not able to do it at all by myself. When people sharing the job work in harmony, any job can be easily done no matter how hard it is. If we cannot make changes out of ten, twenty hours of people who practice with us, the time cannot be turned into creative energy source.

The time and space in Oriental studies are the keys of change. ju-yeok (the Book of Changes) is to study those changes and the nirvana is the Buddhist practice to be freed from the restriction in the time and space. Time matters but you shouldn't be obsessed with the time itself. To get out of the time, you should be able to utilize it by objectifying it. It is the same with people. It is wrong to take advantage of people for my benefit but it is important to make them well display their capability. But it is easier said than done because people do things as they think. It's hard to get things done because people only infuse their thinking to others. To utilize people well, you should watch the situation objectively, without subjective emotions, at a more comfortable condition.

For example, everyone insists that they will save the country and organizations and protect their home in emergency circumstances but we don't know until the situation really happens. It would be challenging but how can we think realistically without being swayed by personal feelings? People who are able to do so only can overcome difficulties. It is the same that we know who should do what kind of work for success. In human relations, positive factors and negative ones always coexist. Conflicts arise where people force others to be like themselves.

So does in our workplace. Teachers should truly think of what members want. To avoid conflicts in pointing out what's wrong, people's acts, not people themselves, should be brought up. To keep a good connection each other, don't try to change others but yourself. You shouldn't expect others' change without yours. Even parents cannot do so. It doesn't exist in the universe at all.

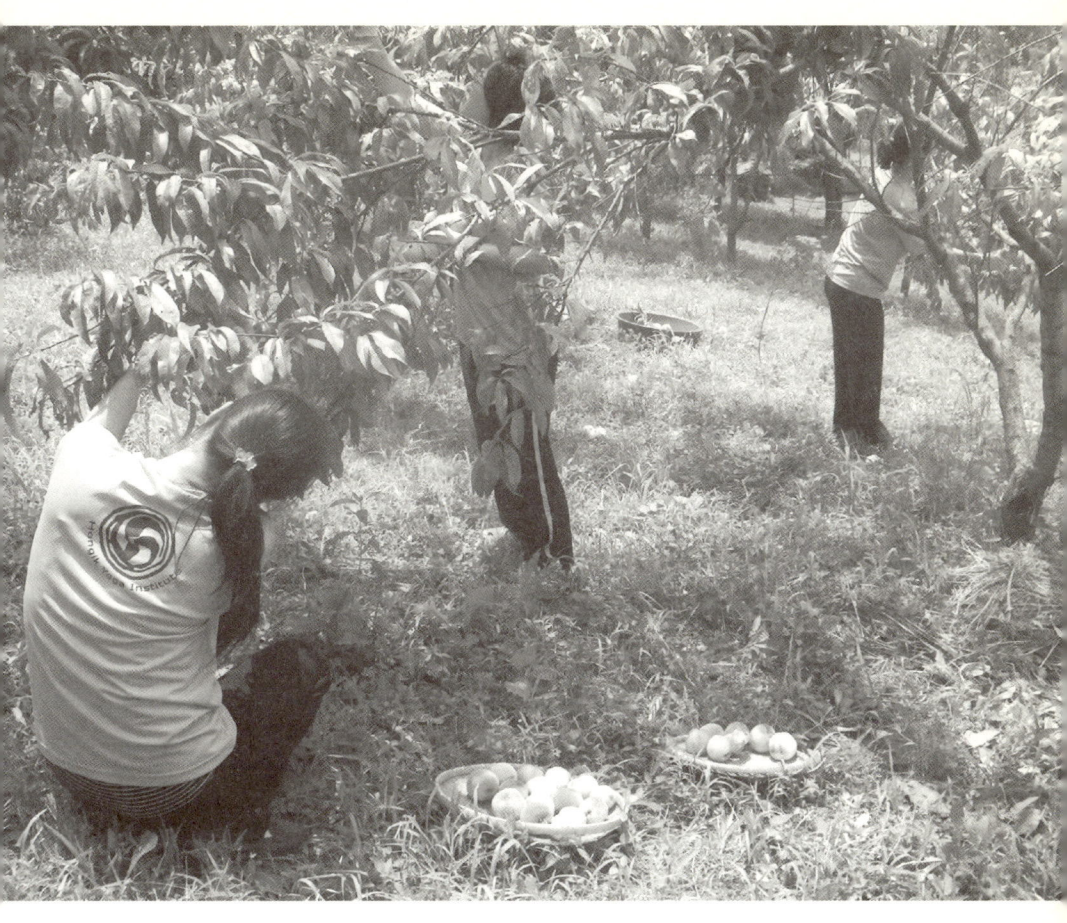

You shouldn't expect others' change without yours.
Even parents cannot do so.
It doesn't exist in the universe at all.

Good Cause and Positive Mind

When we send in positive psychokinesis ourselves, we can cheer ourselves up even in difficult situations and then the positive energies are collected.

No matter how many difficulties people are faced in life, those who are with good cause and belief do not easily give in or collapse. In other words, we do not easily die if we have good cause in doing things. This is what I have certainly experienced and recognized through meditation. Heaven cares for those who follow heaven's will in their lives.

People free from obsessions are given good ideas and inspiration from heaven. Without a heavy mantle of consciousness, everything feels comfortable and looks beautiful. In this respect, the meanings of Yoga Sutra by Patanjali[30] are well delivered only to those who truly want to study yoga. This study should be done heartily. We generally get anxious only about being pissed off, not about seeking clear consciousness.

We don't get unhappy only with positive thinking that life is upon our mind. When we send in positive psychokinesis ourselves, we can cheer ourselves up even in difficult situations and then the positive energies are collected. Only when we have this mind, we can overcome a lot of difficulties coming from the process of practice.

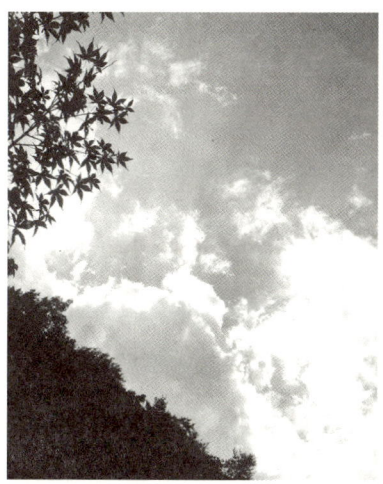

---

30) Theories on him are not united. Even about his birth, it ranges from 900 BC to 300 AD and his birthplace is assumed either as Chidambaram in southern India or as Bengal. However, there are no two ways about it; He is called saint or father of yoga who organized Yoga Sutra whose authority on yoga is well acknowledged.

Ought to Have Spiritual Pride

The border of what I know and what I don't should be concrete.
This is a spiritually important issue.

If you want to live a natural life, you should choose and do what you can do well. If you ask for the moon on what you are not good at, you cannot exercise your capability. As we get energy through sincere prayer when we are distressed and agonized, mantra at the end of our despair becomes our energy and we come to realize that all of knowledge that we used to believe as our assets is not that much useful. Even though we read so many books on philosophy, religion and psychology which deal with truths of life, what would they mean if we cannot recall a single phrase to cheer us up or cannot find anything to put into action in hard circumstances? In this regard, research of knowledge without a sense of purpose cannot be driving force to make changes in life. Therefore, the border of what I know and what I don't should be concrete. This is a spiritually important issue.

We should practice good deeds in our lives. We should change our life energy with positive psychokinesis for lost souls with resentment to go back to where they came from and for everyone to be happy. We won't be totally ruined after experiencing changes in energy. No matter how hard things are going, I believe we will not be that much pathetic. People who aim to live a natural life may not be fancy but be with exuberance. In other words, their lives would be easy. I have never dreamed to be a business tycoon but I didn't set off to get treated to drinks by friends even once in my troubled adolescence. It was because I had my own power of thinking and cause which my meditative life had brought to me. Trained this way, I haven't felt much difficult after getting into my way of yoga and practice. Hunger with good cause never becomes ugly. People who have hunger without good cause study other's face. In addition, those who are with clear philosophy on themselves should have a spiritual pride, not an emotional one.

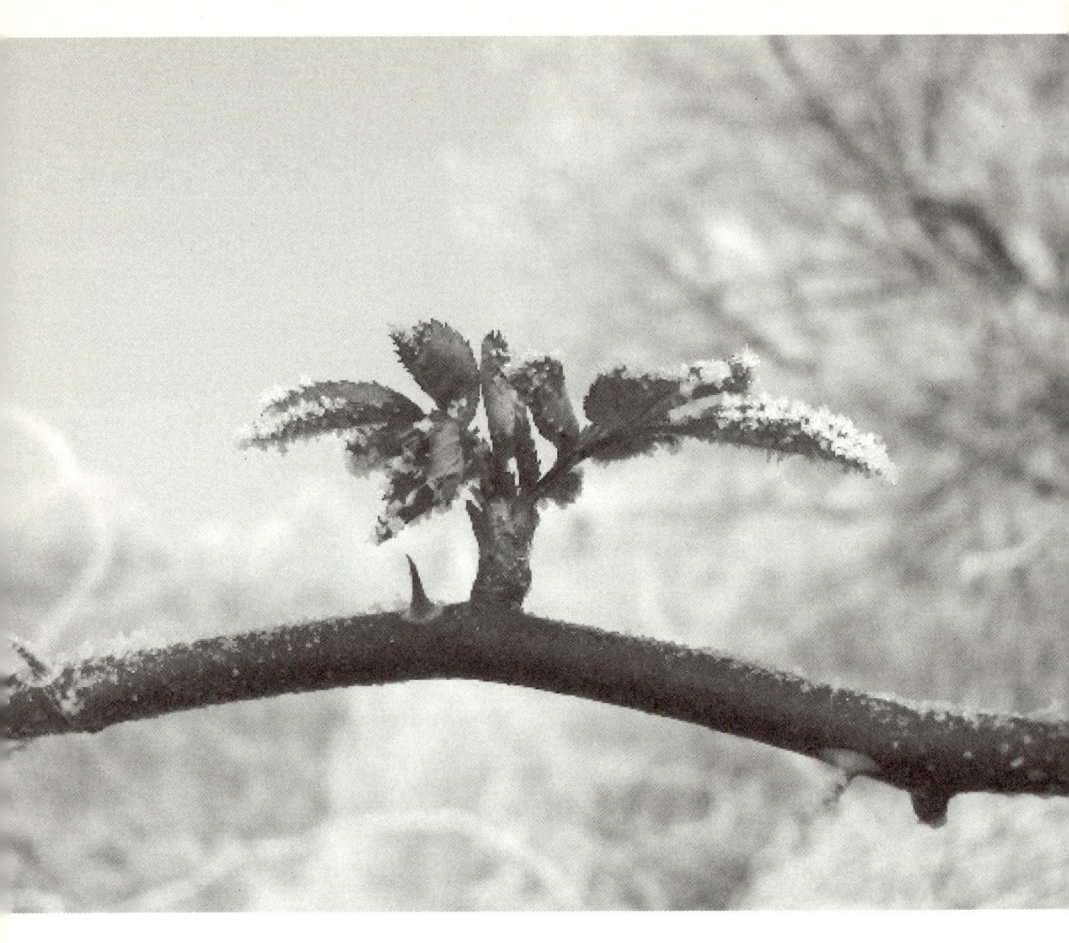

Hunger with good cause never becomes ugly.
People who have hunger without good cause study other's face.
In addition, those who are with clear philosophy on themselves
should have a spiritual pride, not an emotional one.

Devotion only to Shine in Teaching Practice

Teachers should only have shining energy beyond their gender.
I call it 'devotion.'

A large number of yoga teachers have been fostered due to yoga boom of a few years ago. There seemed to be yoga studios in almost all buildings but where have all those studios and teachers gone?

The name of yoga teacher appears strange to me but we are called teachers by members. Members include people of all ages and both sexes and some people have higher status and level of education than us. There are the rich and the poor as well. Some are physically and mentally destroyed while others have clear consciousness.

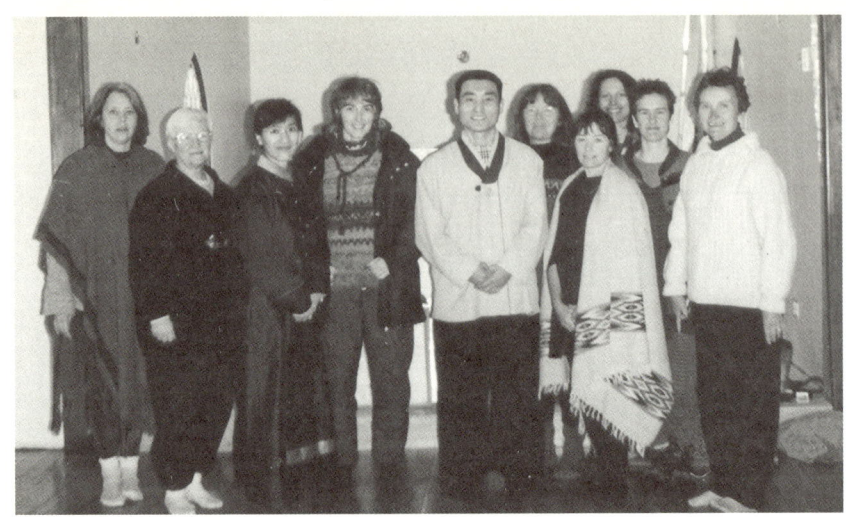

After finishing the Canada workshop

As people do yoga for health and it becomes popular, there also are various side effects. For example, if a business requests a yoga class saying that 'Send us a female teacher if possible,' its intention is generally clear enough. They just want to take a rest and feast their eyes on a pretty woman teacher in good shape for couple of hours rather than truly learn yoga. It is reality.

Female members feel relaxed with a female teacher when they do postures which expose their navel. On the other hand, they may have psychological discomfort if a male teacher comes in when they do vidalasana. What should they do then? But that's not all. Those who are deeply interested in practice itself feel changes in their energy. With these various styles of members in different circumstances, what should we so-called instructors do to be truly called a teacher? Have you ever thought about these things while teaching our members practice? So, teachers should be of the neuter gender. Teachers should only have shining energy beyond their gender. I call it 'devotion.'

We speak out only with devoted practice. A judge speaks with the ruling and a disciplinant should shine only with devotion through practice.

Are You Guys Happy Now?

Not being happy is different from being unhappy.

Along with the current in today's world, you may feel both physically and mentally exhausted but as the saying goes the grass is always greener on the other side of the fence, life is entirely relative. Some living on a mountain miss a city and others worn out in a complex city miss a mountain.

It is impossible to get an answer on a simple valuation basis but a mutual interest of all human beings is to be healthy and happy regardless of their fields of work or conditions where they are put. As you know, we are not truly alive without health no matter how favorable conditions we have. The most important issue in life is upon commonsense truth that you already know of.

Let's talk about happiness. Many philosophers and thinkers define happiness and most people have their own standard of happiness. But most of them say with one voice that happiness is not far away but on their own palms. Yes, they say that happiness is not upon certain circumstances or conditions but in their hands.

Are you guys happy now? Do you have happiness on your palms? As a member of this group, I also ask that of myself. Am I truly happy? This is my answer. My life is not of the supreme happiness but I feel happy for it. The number one reason why I answer it is not of the supreme happiness is that I haven't achieved goals set for this life yet and that I don't think I haven't been earnest in my life to the utmost. Even so, that I feel somewhat happy is because what I have to do is all related to the group and I have found subjects for my study through various human relations great and small. I have those things to study and I do not consider my life boring or listless as I still have energies left for creatively seeking other subjects.

I want to ask people if they are happy. Here are interesting statistics that you might know. The countries with the highest level of happiness are the low-income Bangladesh and Nepal. Even we Koreans enjoy much more material affluence than they do, why are we not happy as they are? My answer is this; we are obsessed with relative things. In other words, when people are asked whether they are happy, they answer they are not happy while thinking that the relative concept of not being happy is just unhappiness. Not being happy is different from being unhappy. It's not true that I am unhappy when I am not happy. Happiness is up to the way I accept that. The key of accepting is self-satisfaction. People who can be self-satisfied do not have greed. Thus, even in doing the same work, some people enjoy the work while some others are obsessed with it. Those who can enjoy the work are not stressed out at least because of the work.

What does it mean to enjoy one's work? To make one's workplace a healthy and happy place, one should have true enlightenment and wisdom on health and should be aware of true meaning and value from happiness. If you guys do more tests on your bodies than I do and you can have a higher and broader standard in the value of happiness, I am sure you are happier and healthier than I am at this very moment. The biggest reason I am telling you this is that you are younger than I. It means you guys have much more time left. So you guys should not ever waste time.

From this time on, you should think that you do your work being free from all thoughts and ideas even in shoveling or cleaning up the trash all day long.

Health and happiness depend upon our mind. Health and happiness are for those who challenge with courage and strong will. Isn't their challenge itself beautiful, sacred and noble? Through thinking bigger from now on, I hope you guys to achieve siddhi[31] in yoga philosophy. Here's a quotation from the Buddhist Priest Sungsan who recently passed away.

Nothing but just doing!

I understand his 'just doing' as doing the best.

Only the best!

---

31) It means 'achievement, completion and success' and it refers to fruits obtained through yoga practice.

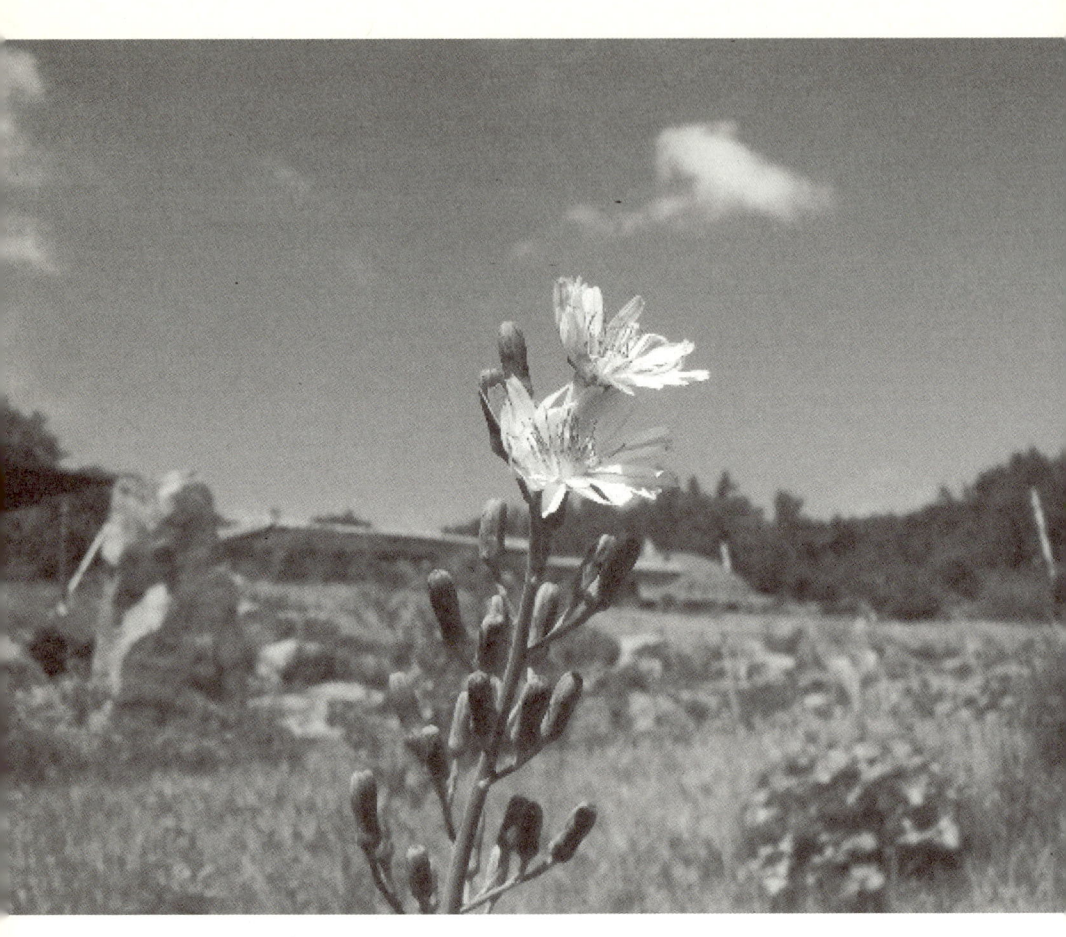

I do not consider my life boring or listless
as I still have energies left
for creatively seeking other subjects.

Katya's Visit to Korea
– Her Spiritual Hometown
– after 10 Years

It is to follow master's lessons as a disciple
and to keep the promise with master.

Even though it's physically far away, I devoutly do mantra and recall master every morning while heading toward east where Korea, my spiritual hometown, lies on with a picture of master, my Guru[32] being placed in practice room at my yoga studio.

For the last few years, people have suggested me several times

---

[32] It means 'a man removing darkness and eliminating shadows' and it refers to a spiritual teacher who gets rid of disciple's ignorance and leads him or her to the path of truth and practice.

to make DVD but I have rejected every single time. It is to follow master's lessons as a disciple and to keep the promise with master. When I left Korea ten years ago, the master said;

"Teach asana only until the time is ripe. You should not teach breathing or meditation clumsily. Only this way, you can protect both yourself and members you teach."

I have sincerely stuck to this promise for ten years and in this context, I've hesitated a lot about making the DVD. It is because I've been well aware that the master hardly makes his appearance in TV or newspaper without a certain principle and he thoroughly sublates the commercial use of yoga.

Last summer, I discussed the DVD matter with master and he allowed me to make DVD during the email correspondence. And I finally came to visit Korea this October in ten years once again with the yoga DVD.

The yoga DVD made this time starts with a dedication to master. It ends with acknowledgement to my family and staff that have helped me, many colleague teachers who assisted my study ten years ago and for the last but not least, the master in particular. The most important point in the DVD is that how my journey to my health, natural life and spiritual exploration began as a yoga disciplinant and where its root was placed.

Over the years after coming back to Canada, I have learned and experienced various styles of yoga from a number of well-known yoga teachers of Canada, America and India. Westerners usually think of 'Indian Guru' to hear about yoga. At first, people were doubtful to see me following an Asian master in Korea which was not even familiar country to them. When master came to visit Canada seven years ago, however, Canadians attending his lecture were so much surprised as he distinctively explained principles of yoga in plain language and they were greatly moved with his passionate energy for devotion to yoga. Even after the workshop, people who were heavily affected by the lecture came to his lodging to ask him questions. His unique way to convey yoga exactly to westerners aroused deep sympathy not only for me but for them.

The master always tells me to ask 'So? Why?' He emphasizes the fact that right understanding and practice of yoga is not two but one. Furthermore, the master confidently said to westerners as this;

"Koreans are nothing without warmheartedness and devotion. Yoga is not about your head but about devotion. Without the devotion, it is nothing no matter how well you do asana and no matter how many theories you've studied."

On this visit, I have my asana tested from master that has been improved for the last ten years and I can study various things about teaching methods for breathing and meditation which I've felt a thirst for. I really appreciate all of that.

It may seem strange for Koreans that a western woman who lives in a faraway country and barely speaks Korean regards this Korean teacher as her master and maintains a spiritual bond even without seeing much of him. As you know well, however, teaching between a teacher and a disciple is not done verbally only. Even at this moment, we are taught by writing and lives of great men and saints in hundreds or even thousands years before whom we've never met. Our hearts are supposed to be of like mind. I didn't know that the relationship with master would be of such importance in my life. However, the more I learn and experience yoga over time, the better I come to understand the meaning. Teachers and members who are directly taught from master and practice with him are so much lucky and blessed.

I love master and all other teachers so much. The 'devotion' in life of Koreans that I have become aware of through master is really beautiful. I will surely get the next meeting not to take this long.

November 2006,
Katya

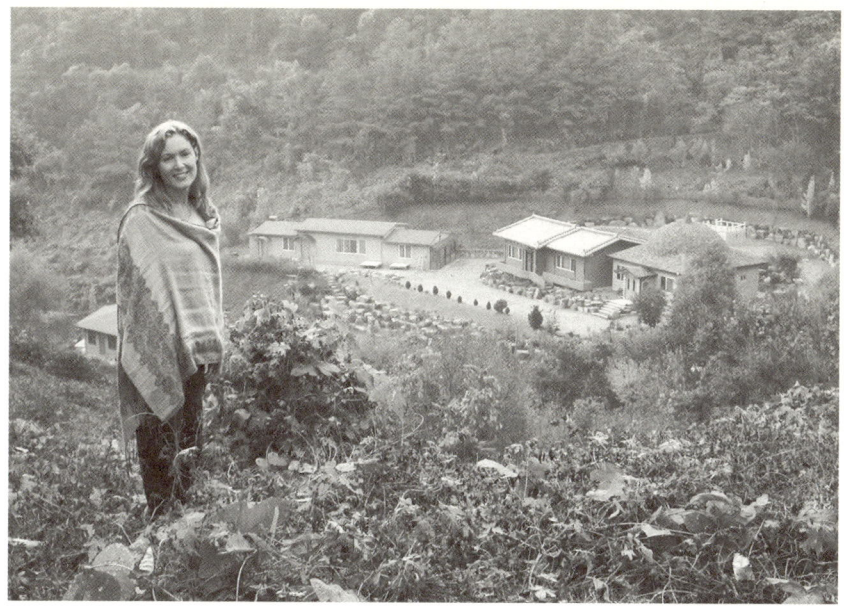

Katya in the interntatioal meditation Center Nae-aneui Ddeul

*Hongik Yoga Institute organized the above based on Katya Hayes' visit to Korea from late October to early November in 2006 to meet up her master, the author, and her stories.

*Katya Hayes : While she lived in Korea ten years ago, she came to visit Hongik Yoga Institute with her husband to relieve stress from living in a foreign country and to practice yoga. She had already had experience of yoga back in Canada and started to study yoga in earnest in Korea with being inspired by practice at the institute and the master Seungyong Lee's teaching method and his lessons. She stayed one more year in Korea and she completed the course for yoga teacher at Hongik Yoga Institute as the first foreigner and left for Canada after obtaining a certificate. She does organic farming in her farm which is a little way off Vancouver and she teaches yoga as well at a yoga studio named "Open Heart." She invited the master Seungyong Lee seven years ago so that he could introduce Korean yoga with Yin-Yang and Five Elements to other Canadians.

The Rain of Your Teachings Still Wet in My Mind

Now I am back in the fullness of family life,
but with the rain of your teachings still wet in my mind
to help me along those difficult moments.

Dear Master,

After a long trip, I am home! It was wonderful to see my children, and to be back into a place of familiarity, but that is balanced with a sorrow from having to leaving Korea.

I had an amazing time with you, and with all the wonderful teachers. I came home so deeply grateful for all that I learned, and all that I felt. 10 years was a long time, but in so many ways Korea was as familiar as if I had been there yesterday. The pervading spirits of the Korean people remain the same, one of peace, compassion, and kindness. Just by witnessing that, I learned a lot. I hope the next time I visit won't be so long!!

Today I was driving to Nelson (about 35 minutes) to teach yoga and I played the mantra CD that you recorded for me. It was so powerful and connected me immediately with you, thank you very much for doing that for me. I will continue to work on it and study it.

Now I am back in the fullness of family life, but with the rain of your teachings still wet in my mind to help me along those difficult moments. I think it will take me a long time to really understand a lot of what you said, but I plan on thinking on it all deeply, and letting it absorb slowly.

Most of all, I want to thank you so very much for all that you did for me while I was there, and also for helping me to get there. All of the lovely food, the ashram visit, the many discussions and mantras, the gift of presents for my family, it all was so lovely, and I feel so grateful for it all. You are by far the most generous person that I have ever met, and by that I learn that giving can be an act of love, and of purity.

When you said that one day you will be an old man in need of care, I smiled inwardly to myself, knowing that one day that will be true and by your side I will sit, as I do now, even if only in spirit.

Many thanks again, and until we meet again, our minds and hearts meet in mantra.

November, 2006
Fondly, Katya

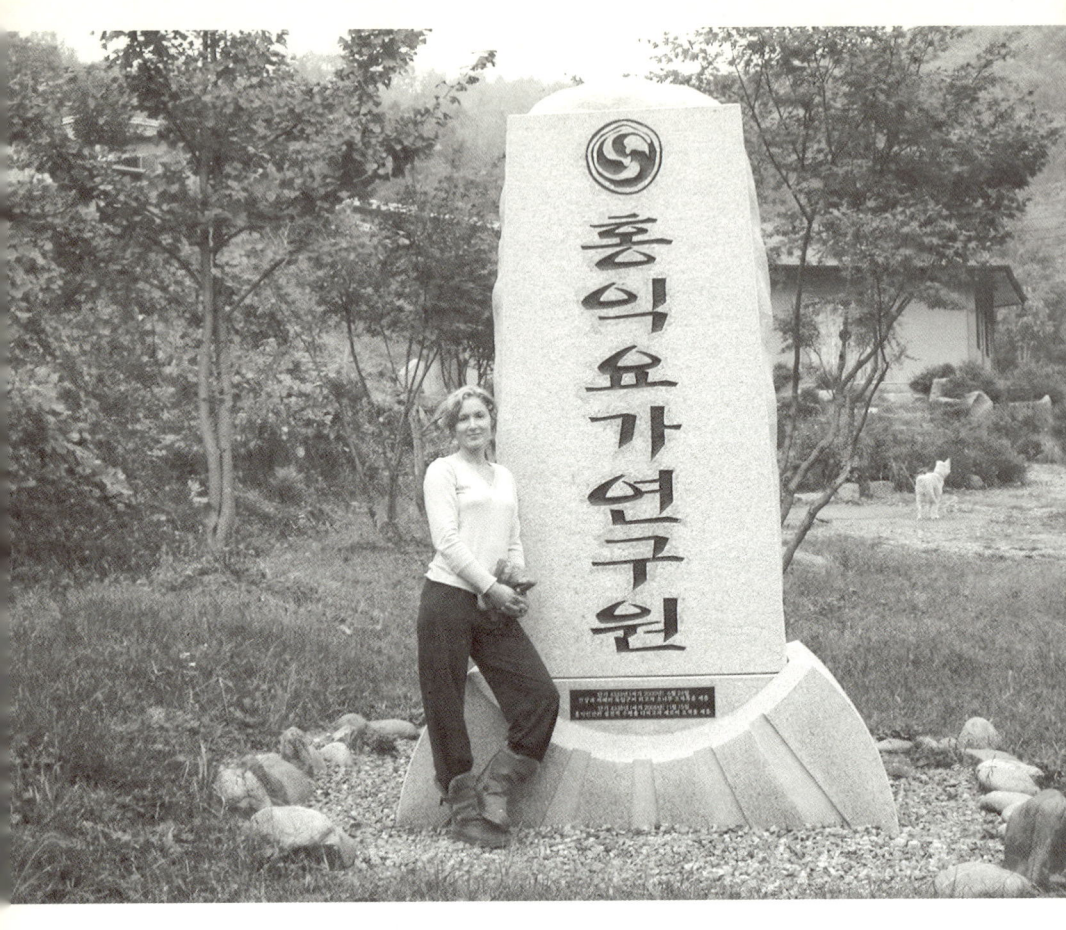

Teaching between a teacher and a disciple
is not done verbally only.

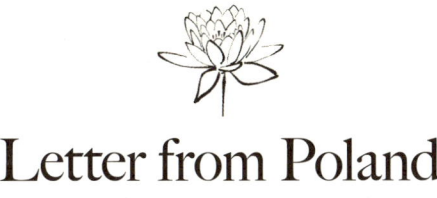

Letter from Poland

Thank you for your good energy.

Dear Teachers,

Please give my warmest regards to Master and Teachers.

I'm sorry I have not written so long, I have some problems with my father, He was at the hospital again. He came back home yesterday. They gave him 5 sessions of radiotherapy (he can't receive a chemotherapy anymore). He feels bad, has a high fever and really strong and frequent hits of coughing. I have been giving him the bamboo salt I received from Master and I hope things will

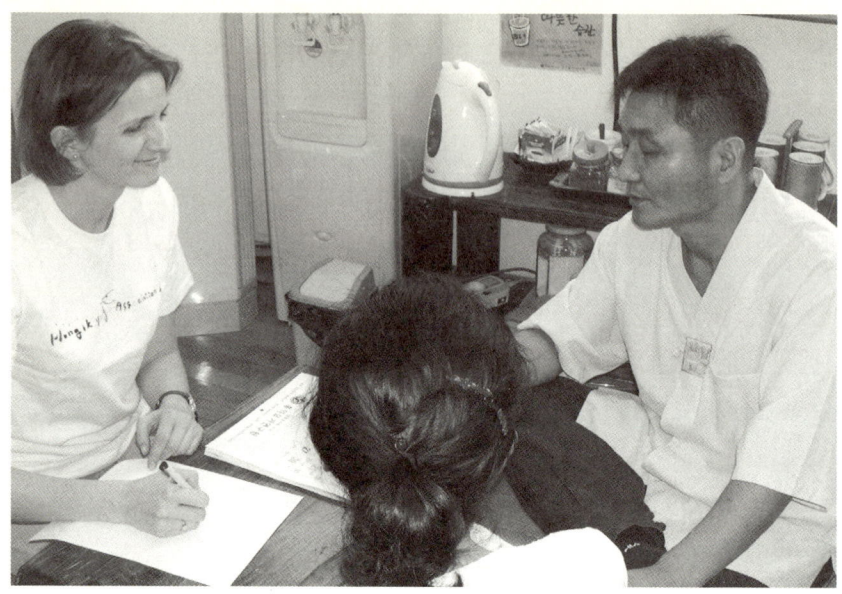

not be worse....

I practice yoga every day at home and I have almost read all the books I received from Master and Teachers. I want to read them again and again more carefully with use of a dictionary and make some more detailed notes.

I can't practice Hongik Yoga mantra because it is too difficult to me now but I started praying as a catholic regularly-in the morning and at night. Thank you for your good energy (I have been crying last month only twice).

We have a difficult situation in my office lately. I must work because I want to live. I would prefer want to work and find in it a sense of life but....

I try to do all the other things making my life good and valuable after work. I try to read in the evenings in a bus or a train and write mails at nights.

Please take care of Yourselves and Your Families and be happy!

The best regards to all members of Hongik Yoga Institute and Hongik Yoga Association.

I hope I will write to you soon. In case you have any questions, enquiries please do not hesitate to write me about them.

November, 2006
Edyta Matejko

PS: Yesterday we had a first snow in Poland. Polish gold autumn have gone away..., till the next coming back after a year.

---

*Edyta Matejko : She studied Korean in Poland, and learned Korean at Yonsei University in Korea.

An American potter came to Korea to learn Korean Onggi
- For a true meditation

Potter should be healthy and potter's mind should be at ease and modest, and then potter can make brilliant vessels.

From the first time I came to Korea to learn Korean Onggi[33] a few years ago and saw the Korean Buddhist monks living in the monasteries. I have been interested in meditation. Somehow I came across yoga. I think it was because it is a way to become healthy and meditate at the same time. Also doing yoga is very simple all you need is your body and your mind. So I purchased

---

33) Onggi is Korean earthenware which is used for storage and utilitarian purposes.

a couple of books on yoga and did it on my own for about 1 year, though not steadily. At first it seemed so logical, but I definitely regret not finding a teacher.

When I came to Korea I was worried that I would not find a place to practice yoga. I am really glad that I was able to find Hongik Yoga Institute as my professor at international language school in Yonsei University introduced me. The asana system is well-rounded, classes on yoga philosophy are offered and there is a very neat diet program. I have been practiced in the Institute and I've got an opportunity to learn Oriental philosophy. Fortunately, I could stay and practice in Kkaedatgi health school which is the ashram of Hongik Yoga Institute. I wrote followings based on what I experienced there for two months.

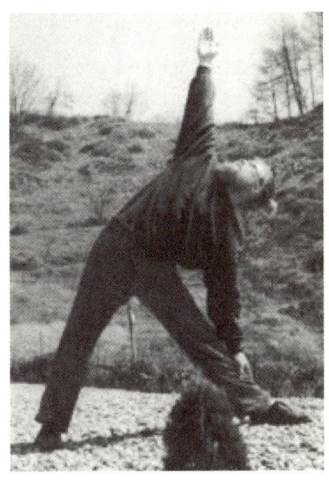

Is it Wednesday or Thursday? I don't notice how time and day passes by nowadays. Since I've been at Bonggol, it passed away half month already. At first there were several people practicing here, so it was interesting to live with them. But at the same time it was difficult to concentrate on practice itself. I've been alone for recent 3 weeks, it's very good but a little bit lonely. Especially when I have meal...

It seems that it has been raining for 3 weeks. The sound that rain makes has been always with me and that natural sound washed away what was in my mind. Now I'm alone. However what is alone is not what is alone. When I am in my room, I fight against flies, when I'm outside, dogs kiss me, mysterious worms, dragonflies, warts, and grasshoppers talk to me.

Over a month I've practiced yoga asana and breathing (pranayama), and my mind became peaceful. Breathing has been improved so much, eyesight and skin also became better. And I myself feel that I became younger 1 or 2 years. With the change of my body, some parts of the body become better and worse repetitively. I think the pain itself is good one because I can get improvement through the very pain. With my mind becoming peaceful, I can breathe better, and I can practice yoga asana with light mind. And I can feel Om mantra practice with my heart. I recognize various agitations in my mind when I can't concentrate on the practice and I see no improvement on it. To practice mind, spirit and body cannot be accomplished without making up my mind stately.

I thought that I knew about practice, meditation and yoga by reading a couple of books. But a few weeks ago, master gave a good scolding to me and said "You don't know." Since that, I started to ask myself even a little about practice meditation and yoga. As time went by I got to realize that I don't know anything as Master said. No matter how much I think, no matter how many books I read, no matter how often I listen to master's lecture, if I don't realize by myself why, how and what to eat, I only keep in believing in other's sayings, that means I don't know anything.

Now I ask only a little and I know I don't know anything. It is sure that person has to breathes, eats and evacuate but I have doubt about what is beyond those categories.

At the first day I came to Bonggol, Baw (a name of Poongsan dog) passed water to my leg. With this he expressed "You are mine." Then I got angry, but now I think Baw kept an eye on me and I think I encountered excellent chance to live here. To live here was sometimes difficult and sometimes easy and sometimes hard and sometimes comfortable. I think it's same wherever I go. That is Yin and Yang.

After 1 week, I will have to go back to US. Precisely 1 year has passed since I came to Korea. My parents want me to continue study. But I think it is more important to learn soil, air, fire, water and Ki as I want to be a good potter. Potter should be healthy and potter's mind should be

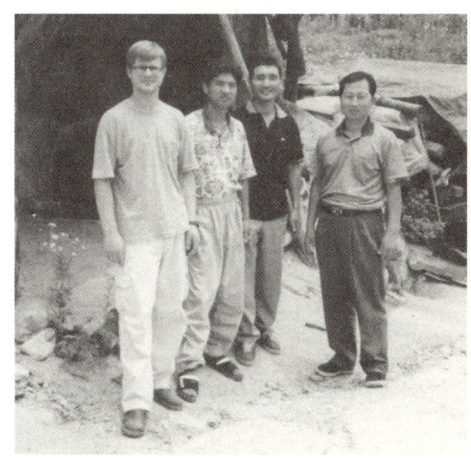

After visiting the traditional Onggi kiln

One Big Desire   179

at ease and modest, through it he can become an ordinary modest potter who puts the whole mind to the work, and then potter can make brilliant vessels(yonggi in Korean).

And I won't forget what master told me. In the day of departure, I tried to make a bow on ceremonial occasions, but master refused it and asked me to ask myself why I should practice and why I've got tied with Onggi and Korea. Why? Why? He asked me to ask myself "deep why?"

Encouraging me to practice hard in US also, Master presented me with grinded Honghwa seeds and ginger tea.

"Yonggi, What do you know? Take out what you know. Yonggi! How can a person who cannot make soil, water, fire and air make ceramic? How!?"

Ask and ask yourself over and over.

September 19th, 2000
Leaving spiritual land, Korea Lee Yonggi

* Lee Yonggi:He majored in ceramic art and he fell in love with Korean Traditional Onggi. His American name is Dustine Whitaker. He practiced in the Institute and ashram in Chungju and went through our national spirit and the wisdom of Oriental philosophy including Yoga. And he decided to practice touching soil all his life and went back to US temporarily in order to prepare a full-scale practice.

　Above writing is written by himself in Korean. Though grammar is partly wrong, it is not corrected so that his feelings are well conveyed. The name of Lee Yonggi is named by himself to express himself as a potter.

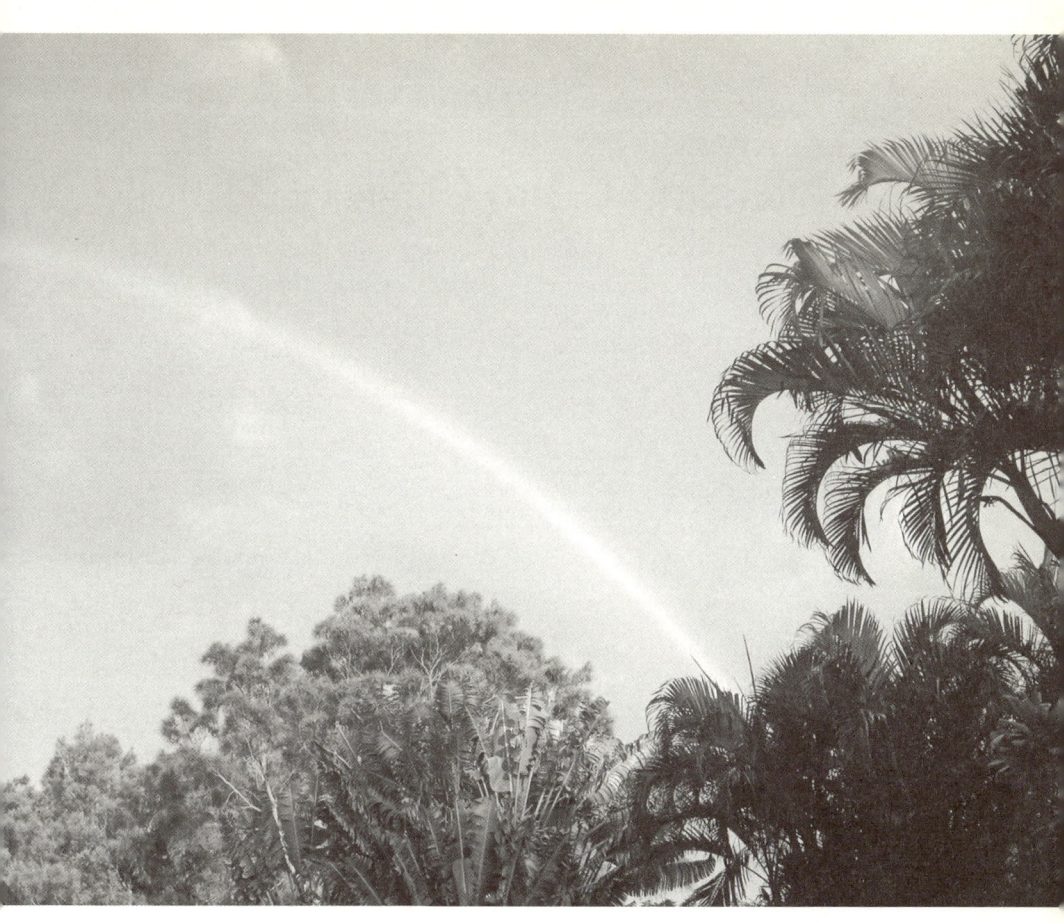

No matter how much I think, no matter how many books I read,
no matter how often I listen to master's lecture, if I don't realize by myself why,
how and what to eat, I only keep in believing in other's sayings,
that means I don't know anything.

Nice and Calm Oasis of Mine

Hongik yoga institute was a nice oasis of calm
where I could come to forget about my exams or papers
and just breathe and stretch

Now that I'm getting ready to leave Korea, I have been thinking about what I will miss when I return home to Britain. The Hongik Yoga Institute is certainly on my list. I have really enjoyed coming to Institute to practice yoga and I hope I will be able to find somewhere that is as open and welcoming so that I can continue practising when I am back at home. First began coming to the Institute in October 1998 because I wanted to do some kind of exercise to keep my body healthy. I had tried yoga once before in Britain, and although it was difficult, I had enjoyed it. So, when

I found the Hongik Yoga Institute, I thought it would be a great place to come and try to reach my goal of keeping fit.

Coming to the Institute has been a constant in my otherwise hectic and changeable lifestyle here in Korea. When I first started yoga I was studying at the Graduate School of International Studies at Yonsei University, Taking Korean classes, and various other things.

My life was very busy, and the yoga institute was a nice oasis of calm where I could come to forget about my exams or papers and just breathe and stretch! It was also a great place for me to practice Korean, especially my listening skills. When I first started yoga I was a little worried by the fact that my Korean language ability was so poor. I thought that I would not be able to follow the instructions and would do some damage to a muscle by stretching or bending the wrong way. However, with the assistance of the yoga instructors and by following the other people in the class, I soon got the hang of it. Now, after more that a year, I am happy to find that I understand a lot of the instructions.

I returned to the Institute after a 3 and a half month break in September 1999. Since that time I have been making every effort to come at least twice a week. And also, since that time, I have become more aware of the benefits of practising yoga to my personal health and mental well-being. In terms of my health, yoga has helped me to stay fit. I have also found that my body has gained more definition as the exercises are now beginning to reshape my waist, hips and legs. Although I still have difficulty doing some of the poses, I think I have become more flexible and can do a lot more of the stretches than when I first began. These days I have to deal with a lot of stress because I am now in my final semester a Yonsei and have to write my graduate thesis. Yoga has helped me to stay calm and focused during this stressful time, for which I am very grateful.

So, to all of the yoga instructors at the Institute, thank you for your teaching and your kindness. I think that you are all very caring and considerate people, and I have really enjoyed taking yoga classes at your Institute. I will take away good memories of practising yoga in Korea. I wish you all continued happiness and success in the future.

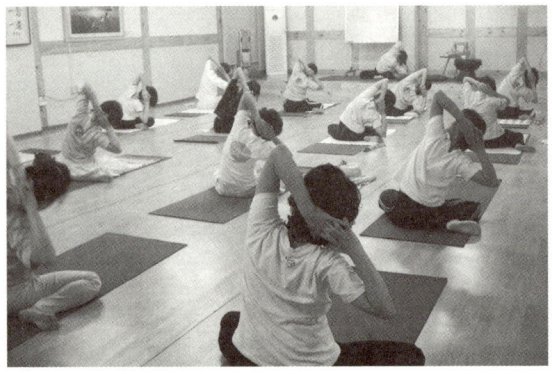

* Deborah Ranger : She majored in international management and business administration in Yonsei University and went back to England.

The Spirit of my Yoga Master

The tree dressed in clothes of Master Lee survived again.

I left Seoul at the end of February because I became a professor of English at Honam University in Kwangju. But before I left Master Lee honored me with a gift of his old hanbok. I knew the gift was special and it was much more than simply a gift of an article of clothing to another person. I felt that wearing it would almost go against the spirit of what the hanbok represented. I wanted to keep the hanbok in the realm that it was presented to me, in the world of the spirit.

Off and on the past twenty years, I have been a sculptor in the

United States. So, I made up my mind to create a sculpture. You must understad that it is not as if I am in my studio in the United States—I had to use whatever is available. During my time in Korea I've noticed a particular tree that people have in their homes and then are thrown out after they die. I saw many of them in Seoul.

What struck me about this tree(I still don't know its name) is that its branches wrapped around each other like snakes and the form produced was similar to the kudalini energy moving up the spine. In Western thought the same shape is referred to as the caduceus and is used as the symbol for medicine. After I moved to Kwangju I picked up one of these trees off the street. The tree appeared completely dead and I took it home and wrapped the hanbok given to me by Master Lee around it. I got a few stones to put around the base of the tree to help hold it up and I gave it the title 'The Spirit of My Yoga Master.' The idea of the title was to honor Master Lee but even more so to honor the lager Spirit which gives our life nourishment and meaning.

The sculpture stood in the one of the rooms in my apartment for several months. And then a strange thing happened. Suddenly, shoots began growing out of the dead tree. I and my wife Ko were a bit shocked. After all, the tree was not even planted in dirt, it was standing on the floor. We had not watered it. Nothing. And yet suddenly several shoots with leaves began growing out of its dry and brittle bark. We were both quite amazed. It is still standing in our apartment and though some of the original shoots and leaves have fallen, new ones have taken their place.

---

* Szaja Gottlieb : He is American sculptor. Two years ago, he had come to Korea for the purpose of studying Oriental thought and art working. Those days, he practiced yoga at this institute. Even though he is older than master, he honors master as his guru (mental teacher) until now.

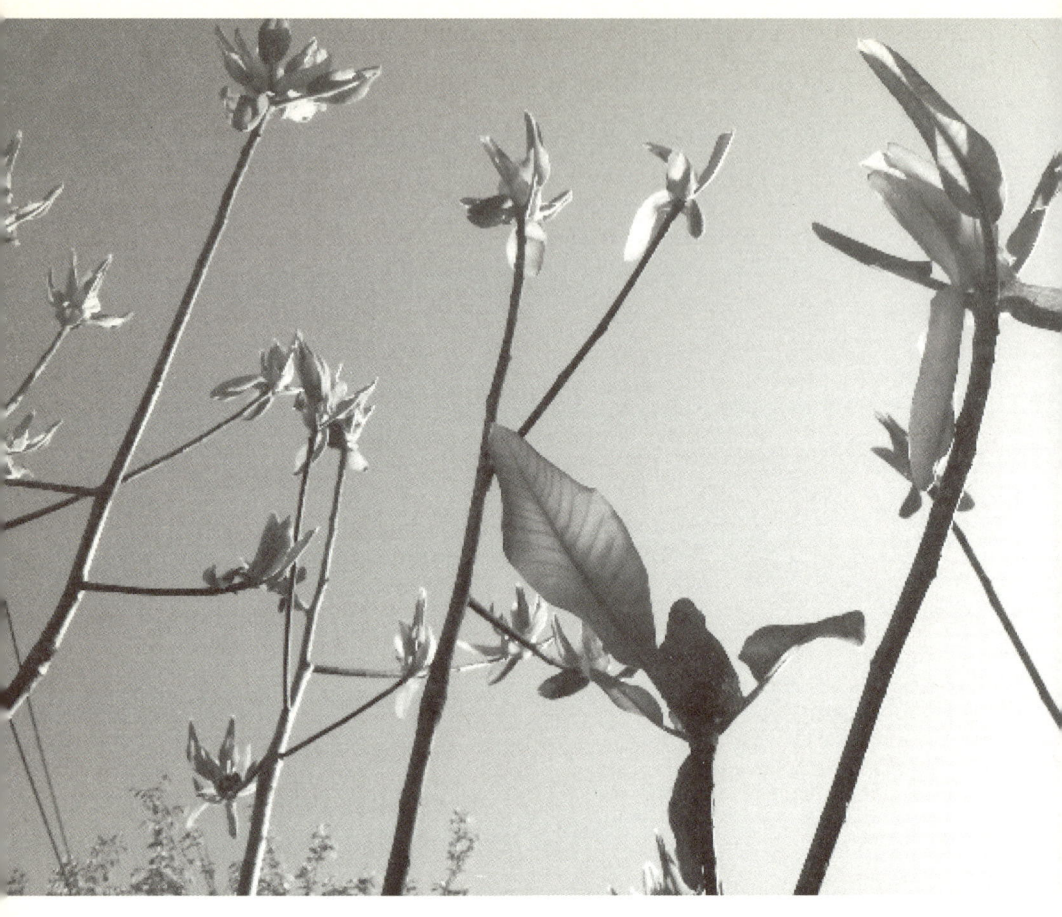

In the nature, human feel true happiness.

After the Hawaii Yoga Training
What I received from the master is more than just materials.

The autumn sky is getting higher. The golden wave of rice in fields is surging with wind and people look a little relaxed and expectant before Han-ga-wi (Korean Thanksgiving Day) in their somewhat hardscrabble life.

When we look around ourselves from time to time, we come to naturally think that so many people live their life to the full working from dawn till dusk in a sweat. We also introspect ourselves recalling monks who would give up pride of life for spiritual enlightenment and who would start a day from early in the morning with their breath.

What I heartily thought at the Hawaii yoga training this summer was that 'Why is my master taking that much difficult path? If he taught westerners like Priest Sungsan, much more disciples than he has now would follow his teaching and he would also be more comfortable.'

We can see this in the well known Priest Sungsan's life story. Sungsan who used to be active in propagating successfully in Korea and Japan went to America where he even couldn't make himself understood in English. What he did for a living was a washing machine repairman It was thanks to the fact that he had attended a technical high school in Pyongyang. His wages would be ridiculously low because he was a foreigner who couldn't speak the language. With a name tag 'Mr. Lee' pinned on his chest and diabetes, his long-lasting disease, he paid his rent and fed his disciples with money earned while breathing in heat of the laundry. It is said that his devoted behaviors of teaching blue-eyed westerners with this hard-earned money and taking care of them seemed miraculous beyond just moving.

For those who earn money from yoga and achieve fame, our master would seem that way as well. What for he gives people such vociferous lectures and scolds people and teach them to eat well and live a good life by traveling through driving down the highway from the early dawn and giving them farm produce that he harvests? And he also tells them to brighten up with eating their fill. That is the elders' love for the young but still, wouldn't we have to devote ourselves with clenched teeth so that our master can focus only on lectures and his teaching?

What I received from the master is more than just materials. As Jesus shared bread and wine while calling them his blood and flesh to his disciples, we received our master's energy and spiritual food. If we couldn't see that, we do not need to be with him to attain Hongik-Ingan through yoga. People say that nobody knows what our relations of today would be like tomorrow. We cannot assure till when we can be together to study and to teach. Who could guarantee that tomorrow will be like today?

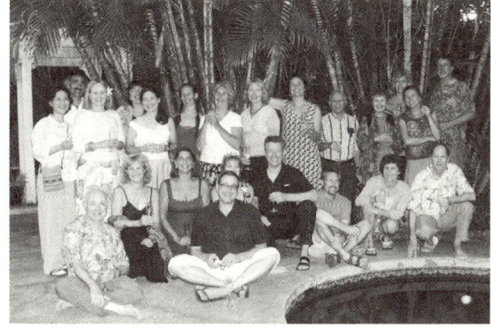

Thus, I think we should beat up ourselves at this very moment that is about to get watchless and lazy and we should also try hard to acknowledge our problems and to solve them even if it hurts. I now look back the moment when I first went into the world of yoga and met my master. Whenever I have problems, I will ask myself patiently over and over for solutions on my own.

September 26th, 2006
Youngse Jang

After the Pilgrimage to Himalayas

Wouldn't I be able to be a better person
after visiting such a huge and sacred place?

Hello, master.

It was just a few days ago but it seems like a faint dream already that you, my colleague disciplinants and I came back from the pilgrimage to Himalayas. I am writing to you looking back on my memories to organize what I felt and studied on my own.

On 25th December in 2006, we headed for Nepal leaving Korean where people were welcoming Christmas. After seven-hour flight, finally in Katmandu, the capital city of Nepal, where there was time difference of three and half hours from Korea! On roads even without the centerline, people, cars, cows, bicycles and dogs passed through all tangled up but to our surprise, no one complained or had an accident. Would it be a little exaggerated that I felt realistic at that moment saying 'I am finally in an exotic foreign land. I'm in Nepal, the country of Gods'?

After unpacking at the hotel, we immediately went to a Buddhist temple instead of looking around streets which had been our original plan. Master told the tour guide to take us to the temple as the beginning of our journey instead of street sightseeing. Even though I didn't know anything like history or reasons of the temple which was colorfully decorated with red and gold with splendid dignity, I could subtly smell the scent of the time with benevolent-looking golden statues of the Buddha which seemed to penetrate our inner side and with monks who drew mandara[34] with colored sand at a corner of the temple. Even for a short prayer, I could feel its piety, which might be like the air in a place of practice accumulated through a very long time. I think everyone would collect their mind straight regardless of their religions.

---

34) It means 'circle' and it is a geometrical figure in which pagods or attributes of God are drawn.

One Big Desire

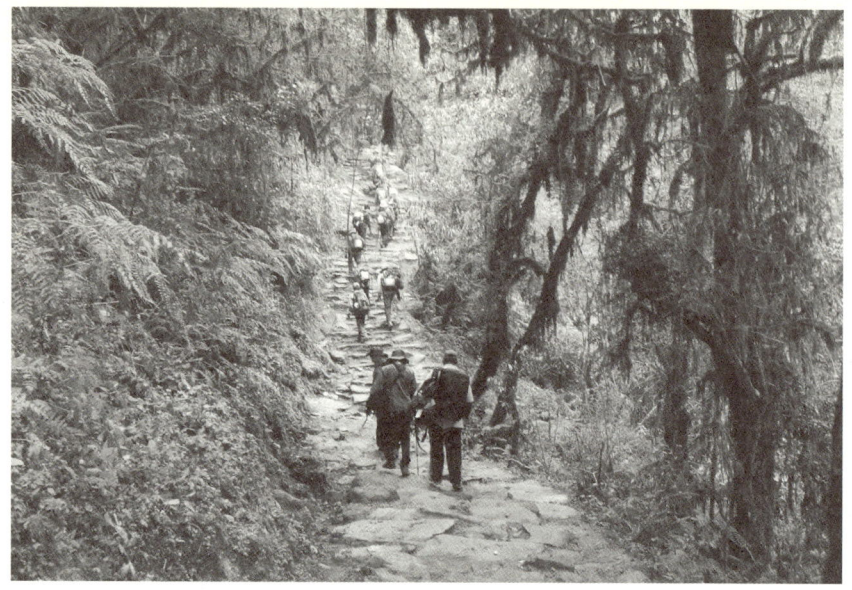

Next day, we left for Pokhara through a domestic flight which was the city where our hiking began. Due to a thick fog, we should wait for hours but later I was told that after the flight we took, there were no flights at all for a few days. I felt sorry for people put on the next flights but we were fortunate.

We again took a bus after the flight for the start point of hiking. Due to the delayed flight, the three-hour hiking planned on that day became so much tight. The sun was going down. We were so busy that we couldn't even catch our breath. We started climbing up and when we were out of breath, the evening set in earnest. That scores of people climbed up rocky hills depending only on a few head lamps was not easy at all. Furthermore, how heavy our loads were! By the time I gasped for breath thinking 'This is really tough,' we barely arrived at the first lodge mountain cabin. Being totally exhausted, I felt a little bit alive after drinking a cup of warmed milk tea.

The first night in Himalayas, we did mantra subsequently after dinner and then tried to sleep in a poorly-made wooden bed with having our heads out in a sleeping bag put on a thin mattress. It was the cold that we couldn't but feel cold even by wearing as many clothes as possible. I fell asleep as shaking to the biting cold. What was strange was that I felt so much cold and tired while my heart was all aflutter. The dawning sky I looked up for a moment at daybreak was all with stars literally seeming to rain in perfect darkness! I feel sorry that I cannot share with others what I saw that day and captured within myself.

The following day, we started mountain climbing, going up and up. I remembered someone saying that it would be leisurely hiking but it was totally mountain field exercise. Of course, Himalayas were not like a hill in the neighborhood but how could it be all about rising up endlessly? The peaks of Annapurna in the distance seemed like a territory of Gods where people dared to reach. Being too much short of breath, we did mantra to ourselves and climbed the mountain bracing ourselves over and over on every single step.

Master's saying 'Drop even the thinking that you are tired' came across my mind. What mattered was the very thinking I was tired. Yes, that was it. It was just a piece of thinking but it was so hard to change my mind. Having miscellaneous thoughts, I felt disgusted about those thoughts endlessly coming to mind even in such a physically challenging situation with being out of breath. Master's teaching that 'At a moment of opening and closing your eyes, get rid of distracting thoughts at once.' I couldn't even imagine how sharp and fierce my mind should be to remove those thoughts. The thoughts like 'I am so out of breath,' 'The loads are too heavy,' or 'I am totally exhausted' made me narrow-minded and gloomy not allowing me to have a little composure.

Those who climbed the mountain hard were not us or a number of climbers to the famous Everest[35] but the natives of Himalayas like Sherpas and Gurungs. While we climbed with the minimum load in a single backpack, they carried our scrips, cutlery, household goods and other equipment by tying them up to their forehead. What they put on their feet was just slippers. Among them, a person a little better off wore sneakers made in

---

[35] It is said that this name is actually not correct. Everest is a name of a western climber and the natives have their own name of 'Chomorungma-the sacred mother' to call it.

India. Toes coming out of slippers were extremely rough and thick. I felt uncomfortable as if I had peeked at one aspect of their tough lives.

How could I express I was so tired to take care of myself only while seeing them running through the mountains like wind in a sweat even with scrips as big as a grownup? When they saw me feel exhausted and said they were OK and would carry my things with a smile from their heart, I couldn't say a word with a lump in the throat.

They earned just a few dollars for that strenuous job. How worth would it be in Korea? It was so strange. Were they kind to us on purpose to make that money? Could a person deliberately smile like that? How many times have I heartily worried about others and smiled to them?

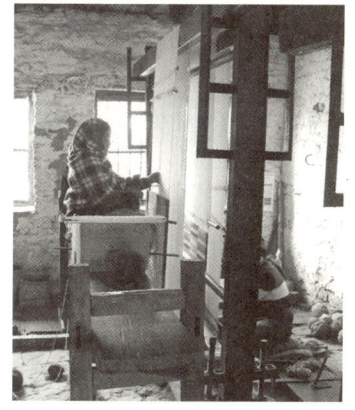

Going up and then down endlessly and then again up unlimitedly. Annapurna hidden behind clouds and fogs turned up for a moment and then disappeared in the clouds. Getting somewhat irritated to it, I couldn't dare to complain that it was so profound and holy even in such a short glance, which might make it the spiritual mountain.

We naturally had difficulties great and small in journey of going up and down. Even heights of 3,450 meter were not considered highlands. As we climbed up higher than Mt. Baekdu, some of us suffered from slight mountain sickness and became exhausted after going up mountains which seemed endless. While supporting and encouraging one another, however, we could safely complete the mountain climbing. Without a number of people who had given a hand, I wouldn't be able to finish the journey. I

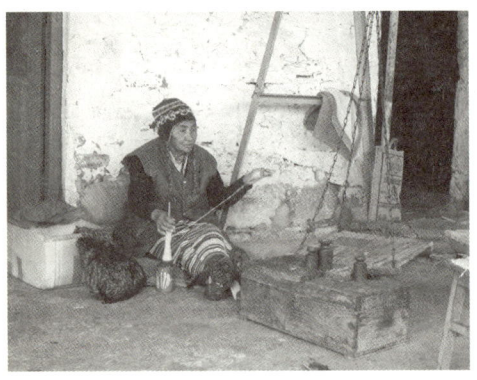

want to express my heartfelt gratitude to them.

For the five days we spent on the mountain, Annapurna didn't completely show us herself. We had some regrets but it would have meant that we should come down there once again. I thought we should accept that way.

Many people I met while climbing – a middle aged woman collecting a purse for her burned house, a middle aged man passing the hat to found a school, children in school uniforms with neatly combed hair running through mountains to go to school which took more than three hours, kids looking at us with a runny nose and bright eyes. Even though they didn't have much possession, their faces were all calm and they seemed not to have ever frowned. It is said that Nepal's level of happiness is ranked the highest all over the world.

In addition, dogs lying to meditate with the most relaxed expressions in the world. As people take after the nature, dogs become similar to the nature and then people living with them. And the Annapurna! We promised to come again someday and came down to the world of human beings.

The most memorable thing during the journey was Tibet refugee town. It was the place where Nepal provided people losing their country with land, houses, carpet factories so that they could work. I was told that money earned through selling the carpet was sent to the Dalai Lama, their spiritual leader. It was a kind of funds for independence fighters. As the master has always told us to be an independence fighter of health and wisdom, we bought some presents there to help raise their funds.

Not only were beautiful carpet and traditional patterns and appearances of Tibetans similar to ours impressive but old ladies spinning thread were so much memorable. Humming 'oṃ maṇi padme hūṃ'[36] to themselves, they were spinning yarn with relaxed looks. Even in my eyes, they seemed to live a life within

---

36) It is representative holy words of Buddhism and it stands for the Buddhist Goddess of Mercy.

practice while I flied into a rage even in practicing after making firm determination of doing mantra, breathing practice or meditation practice. The master's saying of practice in one's living, the practice inseparable from one's life and practice equivalent to life would be like the old ladies' figures.

  I still have so much to tell like sailing on a beautiful lake in Pokhara, the world's biggest Tibetan pagoda with mandala structure on which Buddha's eyes were painted, crematory at Pashupatinath Temple where life and death coexisted, Kumari temple where a living goddess lived, travelers' street in Kathmandu and market places full of colorful stuff and rarities.

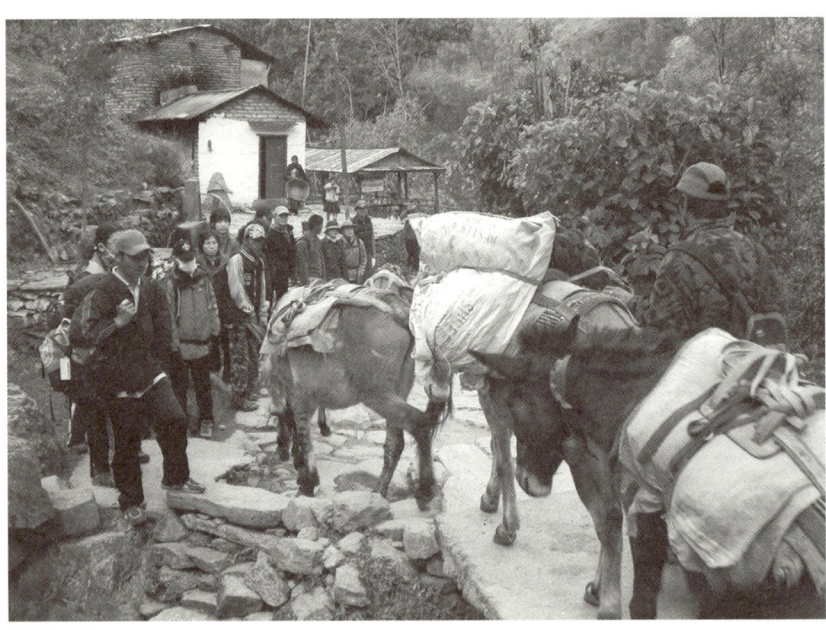

Before heading for Himalayas, I actually had an expectation that 'Wouldn't I be able to be a better person after visiting such a huge and sacred place? Wouldn't it be a kind of inspiration for me?' Thinking it over after coming back, I was like a thief. How can things be changed in a moment after all those years of my life and experiences collected everyday and every single moment? It was nonsense no matter how sacred Himalayas were.

I am blessed enough only with standing before a vast and holy nature, seeing, smelling, listening to and experiencing it. I haven't changed yet for lack of preparation and that may be why Annapurna didn't show up. For me at least.

Mantra. Through this Himalayas training, all of us aimed to do mantra hundred thousand times to humble and purify ourselves but I couldn't accomplish that goal. Due to physical fatigue of being out of breath, feeling heavy for my body and growing weary or the fear and pressure to go down the mountain with endless rocks, I sometimes even forgot to keep mantra. I was all captured by thinking 'Go up. Go down.'

Still, I learned one thing. il-sim (one heart) that I just should go up and il-yeom (one thought) that I just should go down. At the very moment when I couldn't think anything else, I felt that I could walk up the steps anyway. Though this disciple has this small piece of thinking to hit on, the master has raised funds to grant scholarship for this in years past. There's nothing for me to say about it. Thanks to master and so many people and other things invisible, I could make it to Himalayas where otherwise I wouldn't have imagined visiting. I am sorry for your worries on stomachache I had at the last minute and deeply appreciate in many respects. I promise to talk about things untold later.

Thank you, master. Stay healthy.

January, 2007
Jooyeon Park

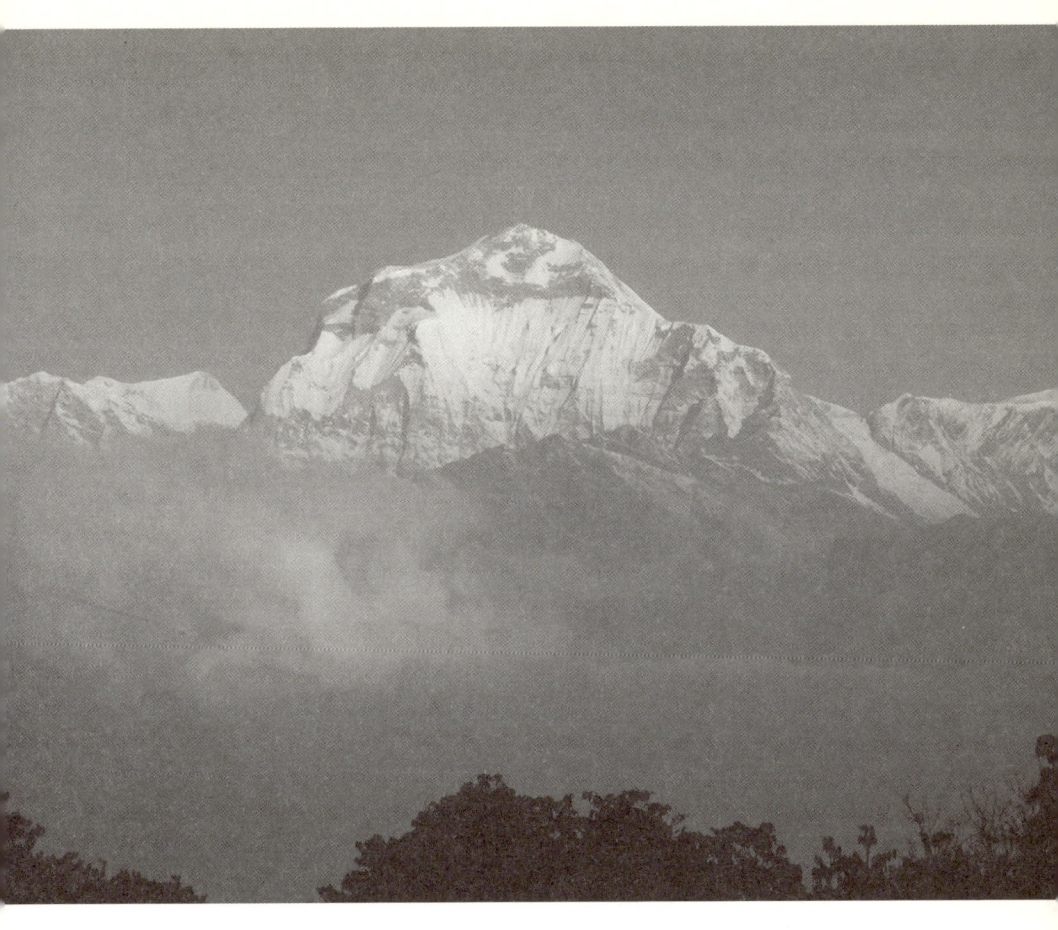

Southern peak of Annapurna in the Himalayas:
Though this disciple has this small piece of thinking to hit on,
the master has raised funds to grant scholarship
for this in years past.

International Meditation Center Nae-aneui Ddeul (Garden inside Me)

International Meditation Center Nae-aneui Ddeul (Garden inside Me) was established jointly by Hongik Yoga Institute and Hongik Yoga Association as the first ashram in Korea. Nae-aneui Ddeul offer meditaion and orthodox yoga practice program, tailored workshops for groups and individuals, knowledge on the proper food and natural health care system based on the spirit of Korea. Nae-aneui Ddeul has red clay meditation room, asana room, Jungwon Natural Health Library, seminar room and accommodations. A lot of people came across Korea and from abroad have spent healthy and true relaxation time here.

By coaching the foreign yoga practitioners and yoga teacher (in Canada and Poland etc.) Nae-aneui Ddeul conveys natural health care system based on the spirit of Korea continuously. We are committed to play a role to create a society together as the cooperation organizations of probation office under the Ministry of Justice and Hue Center of Hankyoreh Newspaper Company.

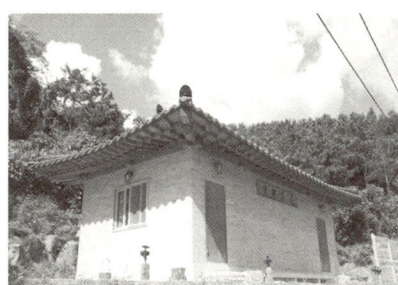
Gabbong-jae (red clay meditation room)

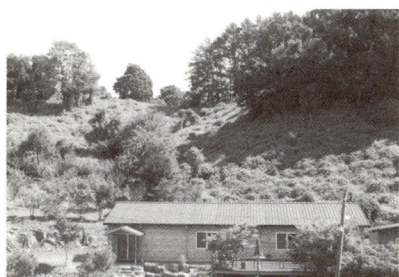
Jungwon Natural Health Library

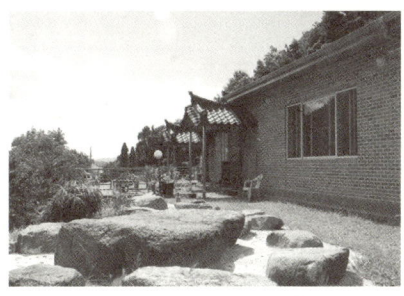
Asanaroom

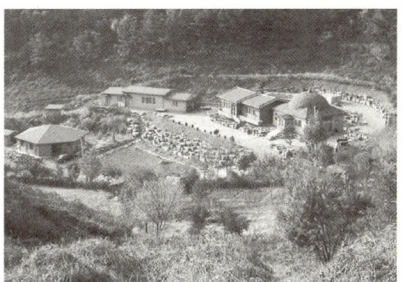
view in autumn

Contact
Address 19, Jodonhandaengigil, Dongryang-myeon,
Chungju-si, Chungcheongbuk-do
Telephone (82-43) 851-1235

Seoul Office_Address 46, Sinchonro, Mapo-gu, Seoul
Telephone (82-2) 333-2350

Email: yogahi@chol.com
Homepage: http://www.yogashram.net